SURVIVING THE
MEDICAL
MELTDOWN

To Sara
For Liberty &
health

SURVIVING THE
MEDICAL MELTDOWN

YOUR GUIDE TO LIVING THROUGH
THE DISASTER OF OBAMACARE

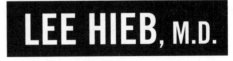
LEE HIEB, M.D.

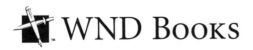
WND Books

SURVIVING THE MEDICAL MELTDOWN

Published by WND Books', Washington, D.C. WND Books is a registered trademark of WorldNetDaily.com, Inc. ("WND")

This book is intended for informational purposes only. It contains general information about medical conditions and treatments and home remedies. Neither the author nor the publisher claims that anything presented is true, accurate, proven, and/or not harmful to your health or well-being. Any information associated with this book should not be considered a substitute for medical advice from a health care professional. If you are experiencing any form of health problems, always consult a doctor before attempting any treatment on your own. Neither the author nor the publisher will be held liable or responsible in any way for any harm, injury, illness, or death that may result from the use of the content herein or anything related to it.

Book designed by Mark Karis. Illustrations by Michael Di Pietro.

WND Books are distributed to the trade by: Midpoint Trade Books, 27 West 20th Street, Suite 1102, New York, New York 10011

WND Books are available at special discounts for bulk purchases.
WND Books also publishes books in electronic formats.
For more information call (541) 474-1776 or visit www.wndbooks.com.

THE HOLY BIBLE, NEW INTERNATIONAL VERSION®, NIV® Copyright © 1973, 1978, 1984, 2011 by Biblica, Inc.™ Used by permission. All rights reserved worldwide.

Hardcover ISBN: 978-1-938067-02-0
eBook ISBN: 978-1-938067-03-7

Library of Congress Cataloging-in-Publication Data

Hieb, Lee D.
  Surviving the medical meltdown : your guide to living through the disaster of Obamacare / Lee Hieb.
     pages cm
  Includes bibliographical references and index.
   ISBN 978-1-938067-02-0 (pbk.)
1. Medical care—United States. 2. Medical policy—United States. 3. Medical economics—United States. I. Title.
  RA395.A3H543 2014
  362.10973—dc23
            2014031613

Printed in the United States of America
15 16 17 18 19 MPV 9 8 7 6 5 4 3 2

To Ernie Rillos, MD, 1956–2009
Former Navy Corpsman, Orthopaedic Surgeon, and Friend

CONTENTS

ACKNOWLEDGMENTS

There are many people who contributed to the writing of this book. Ralph Weber was a great help in understanding and discussing insurance options. The members of the Association of American Physicians and Surgeons, and particularly Dr. Jane Orient, have helped me to appreciate the meaning of individual liberty and the importance of limited government, free markets, and medical ethics. And of course I thank my sons, Mason and Nathan, for their enlightening Socratic discourse.

INTRODUCTION

You may have thought about surviving an economic or political collapse—how you would eat and how you would defend your family and property and things like that. But have you thought of how you would obtain medical care at times of economic collapse?

Over the years, surgeons have traditionally congregated in surgeons' lounges and discussed interesting or difficult cases. In the last decade, I have found my life as a surgeon has changed considerably, and now, while sitting around with my colleagues, I take part in discussions about surviving the bureaucratic nightmare of Obamacare and Medicare, managing our practices to avoid financial collapse, investing in precious metals, buying weapons and ammunition, food storage, and other survival issues. Physicians are smart people, and most of us feel bad times are coming. I have taken steps to move back to my rural hometown, downsize my debt, and relearn some of the self-reliance of my pioneer ancestors. But along with that, I have thought about medical care for my family and myself, and for my community, in times of national crisis.

If we experience the kind of economic collapse experienced by Argentina and Russia in the last decade, Zimbabwe or the Weimar

Republic before that, where will we get medical supplies and expertise? I began thinking of my father's small-town practice and how self-sufficient he was. I thought about my Navy training and experience and the difficulties of rendering emergency medical care in isolated places with minimal supplies and no trained medical specialists for assistance. From that consideration, I have planned for my own and my family's medical security. This book will help you do the same. The goal of this book is to help you to:

1. Recognize the signs of the impending collapse of the medical system.

2. Prepare yourself and others to be as healthy as possible.

3. Be more self-sufficient when medical issues do arise.

4. Learn to navigate the difficult world of health insurance when finding a physician.

5. Create a medical stockpile for times when supplies are not available.

PART 1

THE COMING COLLAPSE

1

HOW WE GOT HERE

America has been the great experiment in individual liberty. Our Declaration of Independence and our Constitution were intended to create a government with one purpose—to safeguard the God-given rights of its citizens. But nearly from the time of this country's founding, certainly in the last one hundred years, Americans have strayed from the principles in those founding documents and have asked the government to do more than protect the rights to life, liberty, and private property—they have asked government to insure their safety.

It seemed innocuous enough at first. Who better than the federal government to keep watch over our food supply? And it makes sense that government requires its citizens to exercise prudent precautions such as wearing seatbelts or motorcycle helmets. Doesn't it?

Well, the problem is that government cannot make us safer, but it can make us infinitely poorer in the attempt. As Thomas Jefferson so presciently opined, "If we can prevent the government from wasting the labors of the people, under the pretense of taking care of them, they must become happy." Although Jefferson had no inkling of Medicare or—God help us—Obamacare, he perfectly described government-run health care in all its ugly forms.

In 1965, Lyndon Johnson, as part of his Great Society programs, instituted Medicare and subsequently Medicaid. Since then, the cost of medical care has skyrocketed, taxpayers have been milked dry, people have become more and more unhappy about the care they receive (we now have a patient bill of rights, not needed before Medicare), and in general, it is harder and harder to get the care we need. Although ignored by the pundits, the reasons are very straightforward once we deconstruct the effect of government on the practice of medicine, which is fundamentally the same as the effect of government on . . . well, anything! Government produces nothing. It only regulates and appropriates.

To get an idea about how government makes everything in medicine scarcer and more expensive, let's look at the pharmaceutical industry. The government does not invent any new medicine; it only makes it harder for others to invent treatments by overregulating researchers. Whereas drugs once were brought to market quickly, limited only by the time it took to do safety studies and marketing (as with each new generation of iPod and iPhone), now it takes on average fifteen years of a major pharmaceutical corporation's time to get through the government morass. That carries a huge price tag. And the delay is not due to more "thoroughness" but to more stultifying paperwork that FDA regulators confuse with actual research and thinking about drug safety and efficacy. Although the proposition is that this makes us safer, consider this: When the FDA says they are saving thirty-five thousand lives this year by passing a new drug, in actuality their institutional stall cost roughly thirteen years times thirty-five thousand lives *not* saved. And if you were a drug executive and your promising new drug hit a snag at the thirteenth year of this nightmarish series of wickets, would you be more or would you be less apt to be honest about the drug's problems? Like a little kid who is too severely punished for a small infraction of the house rules, drug companies are likely to minimize small problems rather than face the loss of fifteen years of financial investment. In a free market, drug companies can quickly assess whether the drug has problems and, if so, move on to a different and better product. And when the FDA denies the sale of a new drug because it is "too similar" to another drug on the market, it is simply insuring one industry's monopoly and denying the opportunity for price controls through competition. If the same oversight given to the pharmaceutical industry were applied to the computer or phone industry, we would be using old, 1950s-style, rotary-dial, plug-in phones, calculators still attached to mainframe computers, and punch-card technology; and they, too, would be overly expensive.

When government pays for something, it regulates. And it regulates. And it regulates. It spawns offices of bureaucrats whose job is to write regulations. The rest of the universe may tend toward entropy, but government by its very nature tends toward more and more organization and detailed regulation. When you go to your doctor or buy insurance, you are paying for the effect of the 150,000-plus pages of Medicare regulation. Your doctor and your hospital or clinic must be in compliance with volumes of Medicare rules or face financial ruin and potential jail time. And of course, you can't get paid by Medicare or insurance companies (who piggyback on Medicare's requirements) without consulting several tomes in order to choose numerical codes for everything you do for a patient. Then, to "prove" you actually saw and treated the patient, you end up writing long-winded, mostly useless (think of those padded essays you wrote in college to get the necessary page length) patient notes that include the bullet points and catchphrases nonmedical bureaucrats use to determine your pay level. For example, if I see you in my office for a fractured leg, it will be difficult (read: impossible) to weigh you because you cannot bear weight on your broken leg. But if you just tell me your weight—accurate or not—I get a point counted toward my payment. Not that your weight has a damn thing to do with my fixing your broken leg, but it is a "fact" that the bean counters at the Center for Medicare and Medicaid services can count. The more beans counted, the more I get paid, whether or not those "beans" bear any relationship to the medical problem at hand. William Bruce Cameron once said, "Not everything that can be counted counts, and not everything that counts can be counted."[1] How true this is. But it is expensive. To be in compliance with the rules, to avoid being charged with a crime, and to get paid, I had an office filled with seven employees and even then hired an external billing service, which took roughly 10 percent of my collected income. Without Medicare, I could have run the office with two employees and no billing service, charging cash at the window, just as generations of physicians did with much lower fees. It is estimated that every time a "third party" is billed, it costs $58 in overhead staff time and paper and fees. And that is a fixed cost regardless of the actual bill, which might have been $20 before all this added expense.

But, you say, aren't the insurance companies and employee-based health plans and lawyers also to blame? Although it is tempting to blame them, and none are truly blameless, they can only function in their current capacity because the strong arm of the government backs up their actions. For example: Why are lawsuits so ubiquitous? Because the average patient has no skin in the game. When patients come to my office, I cannot pass on to them the cost of my malpractice insurance because the government pays me, not the patient. In contrast, when the electric company gets sued for a wrongful death, it can add the cost to your bill. If the problem becomes widespread, it can take actions to make things safer and then alert the public to the *reason* their rates are increasing. In a free market, doctors could post signs in their offices alerting people that they will be charged a surcharge to cover the malpractice costs—just as businesses do with bounced-check charges. And the more government regulators turn out things such as "Guidelines" or "Best Practices," the more fuel lawyers have to sue those who transgress the guidelines.

Companies learn to profit from government overregulation. Years ago, we reused many items in the operating room—drills, Kevlar safety gloves, and external fixators, to name just a few. They could be resterilized and repackaged until they were no longer usable. Then the FDA ruled that if a hospital wanted to reuse items marked for "single use only," it had to submit the results of full FDA-mandated testing to demonstrate that their procedure was safe. Since no hospital could afford to do that level of testing, hospitals stopped reusing items that were marked "single use only." Very quickly, manufacturers responded by labeling nearly everything "single use only"! Thus, the hundred-dollar, perfectly sharp drill bit with one minor moment of use is discarded, as is the five-thousand-dollar external fixator (which does not go inside the body) that could have been refurbished and resterilized for use on many patients.

And the real kicker is this: for all the expense, we are getting less value. The truth is, government health care has never, ever, in the history of the world, anywhere, delivered the same quality of medical care as has the free market. Nor does it care as well for the poor—no matter the shrill voices of the media and academicians calling for government-run medicine precisely for this reason. Soviet medicine was free, universal, and lousy. There were dead cats lying in hospitals—hospitals that had no running water but many HIV-contaminated needles. The only real care was in the black market or at special hospitals reserved for the politburo and high officials. (See appendix A for references on government health care.) Sadly, as we have lost the battle for the free market in health care today, we are traveling along the path to a centrally controlled, Soviet-style system.

The World Health Organization loves to devalue American medicine, ranking it thirty-seventh in the world, somewhere behind Sudan. But in spite of this report card, the powerful and wealthy, when sick, flock to America for care. Boris Yeltsin underwent heart surgery in a special politiburo-only hospital, by American-trained surgeons, and imported Dr. Michael Debakey from Texas to supervise. His free, universal, Soviet health care system was okay for his gray masses, but not for him. Two premiers of Canada and at least one member of Parliament have crossed our northern border clandestinely to get their health care here. And recently the former head of the Canadian health system jumped the border for care. If universal government medicine were so great, why didn't they stay home? When the former Sultan of Brunei needed care, did he go to Sweden or France or any other socialized, "equitable," and more highly World Health Organization (WHO)–ranked country? No, he came here. People who know, and can afford to, vote on quality with their feet. And for good reason. They know that "fairness of distribution," one of the major determinants of the WHO ranking, doesn't really count when you are sick.

What really counts is outcomes. The British journal of cancer, *Lancet Oncology,* in 2007 looked at the survival from cancer around the world by country. On every chart, for every cancer examined, the best outcome, the best survival rate, was in America. And the differences were not trivial. For example, if one considers cancers that affect men, and lump all cancers into a pool of outcomes, your chance of living five years after diagnosis in America was 66 percent, but in Europe it was 47 percent, and in Britain (nicknamed the "sick man of Europe") 45 percent. Canada fared only a little better at 53 percent, which may explain the tendency of some Canadians to jump the border to America for treatment. Breast cancer, same outcome: 90.5 percent five-year survival in America, 78.5 percent survival in Britain.[2] Similarly, you can look at outcomes for other issues, such as deaths after heart attacks or survival of strokes, and again we fare better than the Brits or Canadians with their universal health care. So, in answer to "Who you gonna call?" when you get sick, the answer is "the United States."

Why is there a 20 percent better cancer survival rate in America? A major reason for this discrepancy is the lack of access to specialty care in government-run systems. In addition to the one million–plus patients waiting for surgery under the National Health Service in Britain, many more wait for evaluation for cancer or heart disease. The average time from diagnosis of breast cancer to seeing a cancer specialist in Canada is forty-five days. In fact, only 50 percent of women biopsied for abnormal screening mammography get their diagnosis within seven weeks.[3] In America, we worry if we can't get a patient into the oncologist over a long weekend. My friend, a former oncologist from MD Anderson Cancer Center in Texas, on a family visit to Sweden, visited a local, small-city Swedish oncologist. My friend was over sixty years old and was still seeing sometimes fifty patients a day in America. But the young Swedish oncologist was very different. His office waiting room was packed with patients, some of whom had traveled two hundred miles to see him on the first-come, first-served basis such offices in Sweden use. But at 1 p.m., after seeing about twelve patients, he closed his doors, and everyone still waiting would simply have to come back in the morning. Why? Because the Swedish government health system paid him for only twelve patients, so that's precisely how many he saw.

For every one million people in America, one thousand are receiving dialysis. In Europe it is 537 per million, and in England, 328 per million. Those untreated suffer and die. As reported in a study by the National Kidney Research Fund and Sheffield University, "If the doctors responsible for those patients cannot find a unit to take them, then the only option is for the doctors to keep them comfortable in hospital until they die."[4] And while American cardiologists debate the best noninvasive ways to stratify cardiac risk in asymptomatic patients, Canadian medical journals publish articles concerning the best way to keep people from dropping over dead while waiting in line for care.[5]

But we are rapidly converting our health care system to a European/Canadian model. Already Medicare is denying care (read: rationing) and paying physicians and hospitals at levels that decrease their willingness to take on more or sick patients. The father of the vice president of my hospital needed a special form of pacemaker. He was having intermittent heart arrhythmias (rhythm problems) and was at risk of sudden death. Medicare denied the pacemaker because his "cardiac output" was too high. Now, any physician knows that cardiac output measured during the normal times between arrhythmias will be normal. Cardiac output applies only for chronic arrhythmia, not intermittent, but government bureaucrats without any medical training can't know that. In spite of pleas from several cardiologists, he remains untreated. And since Medicare pays for the service in general, the Medicare recipient is prohibited from paying cash out of his own pocket to any doctor or hospital that accepts Medicare. His only option is to go overseas or wait to die. To government statisticians, death is the cheaper alternative.

If you want a glimpse into government-run health care American style, just look at the Veterans Administration (VA). My friend was a nurse practitioner at a VA clinic a decade ago. She saw a patient who, two weeks previously, had undergone a total knee replacement at a VA hospital several hours away. The patient complained of increasing redness, warmth, and swelling of the knee—signs of a possible post-operative infection. Knowing that infections in total joints are very serious, she tried to get him back to the VA hospital for urgent follow-up care. She was unable to get an appointment without violating standard appointment protocol, but she finally got him an appointment for two weeks later. (In civilian practice such a swollen red joint would be evaluated emergently—generally within hours—by an orthopaedic surgeon.) After being shuttled nearly five hours on the VA van and after waiting two weeks, the patient arrived at the VA hospital only to be told he had no appointment. The appointment he had been given was for *the following year.* I don't know the clinical outcome in this case, but my nurse practitioner friend was disciplined for violating VA protocol, and she subsequently quit. I'm sure someone got a pat on the back or monetary reward for rigorous uniformity of scheduling or some such nonsense.

The Veterans Administration (VA) has had problems since its inception. Congress sought care for WWI veterans and created the Veterans Bureau. The bureau lasted a whopping nine years before being dissolved because of rampant corruption. The Veterans Administration was created to supplant the bureau in 1930, but the VA was in trouble from its inception, at one point spectacularly protested by veterans over pay.

In 1945 the VA head administrator resigned amid accusations of substandard medical care at the VA hospitals.

It seems nothing much has changed. At present, the VA medical system remains a top heavy, bureaucratic, corrupt organization where lip service is given to quality medical care, but medical care takes a backseat to self-sustaining paperwork that ensures bonuses for VA administrators.

Problems range from contaminated colonoscopic equipment to misidentified graves. As reported by CNN, "At least 40 veterans died while waiting for appointments to see a doctor at the Phoenix Veterans Affairs Health Care system. . . . The patients were on a secret list designed to hide lengthy delays from VA officials in Washington, according to a recently retired VA doctor and several high-level sources."[6] Veterans were waiting futilely in line for care while records were fudged so performance bonuses could be paid.[7] Administrators benefitted from shorter "average waiting times," so that's what they got—truth be damned. [8]

There are various reasons for the failure of the VA to give quality medical care, but the truth is that no one cares more about your health than a *private physician* whom you pay directly, who knows you and your family, and who took his/her Hippocratic oath seriously. Hippocrates taught that "Whatever houses I may visit, I will come for the benefit of the sick, remaining free of all intentional injustice, of all mischief." Hippocrates knew nothing about Medicare or the VA, but he knew that there would always be those "third parties" who would be whispering into the doctor's ear, but who might have an agenda other than the health of the patient. A wife might want the patient dead to get his estate. A neighbor might want him dead to scoop up his wife. Government might want him dead to save money. In the case of the VA, the government administrators chose between giving themselves bonuses or upgrading an operative suite, adding physicians to deal with the backlog or providing better pharmacy services. Private physicians are not perfect. They may not always know the right answers. But with rare exception, they are really committed to seeing their patients do well.

Government-run health care cannot be fixed by new administrators or by tweaking the system, because it is flawed in its very definition. Government makes budgetary decisions that determine who gets what, and in the case of medical care, government bureaucrats see medical care as simply a negative cypher on the financial bottom line.

THE FUTURE OF MEDICINE IN THE UNITED STATES

If you are reading this book, you are wisely concerned about your ability to get medical care in the future. Oh, you may be signed up to this or that health plan, or you may get your medical care through some government agency, for example Medicare or the VA. But you are smart enough to realize that having an insurance card in your wallet does not necessarily get you a doctor when you need one, nor does it magically produce the medicine you need.

You may or may not be aware of the first cracks appearing in the system. Like cracks in the fuselage of an aircraft that can be detected only by X-ray, there are certain telltale signs occurring in medicine today that presage catastrophic failure.

- Shortages of everyday supplies are occurring: tetanus toxoid, Valium, propofol, Levaquin, thyroid, other common drugs, and standard items of medical equipment are not always available.

- Wait times for routine specialty care are dramatically increasing; it is not unusual in some areas to wait six to nine months for an appointment with a rheumatologist or spinal surgeon.

- There are not enough specialists to cover emergency room calls.

- Hospitals in inner cities or poorer regions around the country are closing their doors rather than face economic ruin.

- It is difficult in some areas to find a primary care physician, especially for Medicare or Medicaid patients.

- Physicians are becoming shift workers, working for hospitals and clinics, and in the process are contributing fewer man-hours to patient care and are worsening the maldistribution of physicians.

- Insurance companies, facing a business death spiral, are consolidating into bigger and bigger entities that insure fewer and fewer people for higher and higher prices.

No one can predict the day things will really go bad. It is possible that the decline will be quite gradual, with slow implementation of a Canadian-style universal health care system. In Canada, at first nothing much was different, until doctors and hospitals began responding to the perverse incentives in the system. Today it may take a Canadian six to nine months to get a CT scan, and two to three years to find a primary care physician. But since the decline has been very gradual, a younger generation has grown up expecting nothing more.

Some degree of gradual decline is happening now, and it will continue. But I believe that a catastrophic collapse will at some point befall us. This may occur in conjunction with a monetary collapse similar to the recent hyperinflation in Argentina. In this scenario farmers could still grow food and doctors could still practice medicine, but because the fiat currency has become essentially worthless, there is no easy way of exchanging goods and services. In modern history, during this kind of monetary collapse—witness Germany, Zimbabwe, Russia, and Argentina—the average time for real chaos was three to six months. But after a period of time, with barter and with issuing of a new currency, goods and services once again begin to flow. A worse and longer-lasting scenario is a "doctor death spiral."

Catastrophic collapse due to a "doctor death spiral" will occur when we drop below a critical number of practicing physicians. As our population ages, it requires more physician man-hours of medical care. But as our population ages, so too do our physicians. More than half of the surgeons who cover emergency rooms are over fifty. And although they are some of the most productive physicians, they are being overloaded and overstressed, and are beginning to burn out. Many are retiring early; others are dramatically reducing their patient loads. Recent surveys suggest up to 60 percent of physicians are preparing to do one or the other within two years.[9] And the worsening conditions have lead to an increase in physician suicide. At present, we physicians have the highest suicide rate of any profession. "We lose over four hundred doctors a year"—the equivalent of an entire medical school each year.[10] In areas where fewer and fewer physicians remain, it is very difficult to recruit new physicians to the job—since the new docs do not want to be forced to cover impossible patient loads. Around the country, there are already these medical "black holes"—areas without coverage for certain specialties. These areas are enlarging and are likely to become much larger in the next five years.

The one certainty? Things will be getting much worse because the current system is unsustainable—either in manpower or in dollars and cents. And in any of these scenarios, you will need to be medically prepared. That's why I wrote this book. If you want to prepare yourself and your family to deal with—or better, prevent—a multitude of health care issues, keep reading. Forget what you have been told about preventive care. "Preventive care" government-style is *not* preventive care.

The information you will read in the pages ahead will help you negotiate the crazy medical world of today. We will talk about insurance purchasing, getting the most from your doctor's visit, avoiding damaging foods and toxins, and more. But ultimately, you need to be prepared for a future where immediate access to the modern medical care of today is simply not available.

2

THE COMING DOCTOR SHORTAGE

I practiced in Yuma, Arizona, for more than fifteen years. When I first started in 1995, Yuma had become the third-fastest-growing community in America. The hospital was expanding to meet the demand and was recruiting doctors to the community in nearly all specialties. In 1995, these doctors were all self-employed individually or in groups, but all were in "private practice." I was recruited to practice alongside two other orthopaedic surgeons, one of whom was near retirement age.[1] It was hard work and long hours, because we were covering nearly twice the population of the average orthopaedist. But we were able to recruit other young surgeons, and for a few years things got better. In spite of retirements and surgeons dropping off the ER call schedule as they got older, we had decent—if still too busy—practices, and some time off.

But things changed. ER call became worse, with more high-level trauma from extreme sports, and gunshot wounds became more common. Concurrently, the Center for Medicare Services dropped physician reimbursement over 30 percent and tacked on pages and pages of regulations, vastly increasing the paperwork required to get paid. The mobile elderly retirees who wanted to get out of the cold winters came south as "snowbirds" until 75 percent of my practice was Medicare. And the government, in the form of Tricare (military) and Medicaid, filled most of the remaining percentage, until 90-plus percent of my practice and that of my colleagues was government funded. Less than 10 percent of patients had private insurance.

Here's what that meant financially: whereas private insurance might pay the surgeon $4,500 for a spinal surgery (my specialty), Medicare paid less than $1,200. Now, that may seem like a lot of money, but consider that this fee covers ninety days of care in addition to the surgery, and every year I paid $60,000 in malpractice insurance mandated by the hospital and insurance companies. Additionally, the government took approximately 50 percent in taxes. In other words, I had to do forty to fifty spinal operations *just to pay my malpractice insurance* and still would not have paid myself, my staff, my electric bill, my rent, my taxes, and every other aspect of overhead in running a small business.

As government reimbursement dropped and more and more patients were covered by some form of government "insurance," smart doctors moved to cities filled with private-pay patients. It became impossible to recruit new, young orthopaedic surgeons to our area. After all, why work in a town with 75 percent Medicare payment when you could do the same work for over twice the reimbursement elsewhere? Why ruin your health and personal life spending all night in the operating room, taking care of high-level trauma—often with no pay? As the town continued to boom, the need for trauma surgeons and general orthopaedic care increased at a time when we were losing surgeons. In general medicine and other areas, hospital on-call nights were so brutal—keeping doctors up all night in spite of working all the next day—that all the doctors who could function outside the hospital chose to leave the hospital staff for purely outpatient practices. Those who could afford to retire did so. And in orthopaedics, we were left with four surgeons doing the work that was being done elsewhere by ten or more. The hospital demanded 24/7 coverage, regardless of the burden on the physicians, and did not appreciate the impending collapse of the department, in spite of warnings we issued.

At that point, I was fifty-five and could no longer handle eighty-to-one-hundred-hour weeks. I could no longer stay up all night taking care of dune buggy open fractures and then do high-level spinal surgery all the next day. I resigned, which left only three remaining surgeons. Within six months, a fifty-three-year-old overworked former colleague died, then leaving two surgeons, one over fifty-five.

The hospital finally stepped in and hired a hospital-based orthopaedic traumatologist, at great expense. It also contracted with a group from Phoenix to cover night call. But who knows how long this type of arrangement will be possible, as even big cities are feeling the pinch of too few and aging surgeons.

This is my very personal example of a "business death spiral" applied to medicine. At some point, with too few doctors and too much work, the prospects for recruitment of physicians to resolve the problem became slim. You would think that doctors—eager to make a living—would gravitate to where there *was* a lot of work. After all, in the past it was desirable to grow your practice. But the point is not to be busy but to be profitable. In the old days, the busier you were, the more you worked, the more money you made—like any other *real job*. But not so today, where the government tells you what you will be paid regardless of the cost of your overhead. Between 1996 and 2003, doctors who saw increasing numbers of patients would nevertheless see a decline in income. Medicare and Medicaid paid less and less, and the cost of doing business became more and more expensive as the government added thousands of pages of regulation. Today there are more than 150,000 pages of Medicare regulation, and these regulations, although not written by an elected official (a highly unconstitutional situation), carry the force of law. So, in addition to getting paid less and less, doctors have the increasing likelihood of being prosecuted under Medicare fraud and abuse statutes.

To understand how horrible this threat is, first you must understand the insane world of Medicare coding. In the old days when my father saw a patient in his clinic, he charged cash, and for the most part the patient paid him on the spot. (In 1970 he charged three dollars for an office visit, and six dollars for a house call.) He wrote a single-line office note on a large index card, and thirty years of his practice records fit in three drawers of a standard-sized filing cabinet. Today when I see a patient, I must consult a two-inch-thick CPT book and choose a code that describes my care. In the office I must choose the "level" of coding that is determined by a host of mostly subjective factors—how long I saw the patient, how "complex" the patient's problem was, whether I took his or her blood pressure, etc. Then I must dictate an extensive note detailing all these "bullet points" and submit it to Medicare in order to get paid for the care.

Now, there is no way to win at this. I may think a knee pain evaluation is easy because I am an orthopaedic surgeon, while my friend the family practice physician may think such a workup complicated. But we use the same rules for coding, so on the same scale of coding, he will choose a higher level than I do. Who is correct? Well, you cannot be correct. If I do a new procedure for which no code exists, I am instructed to choose the closest code. But a Medicare bureaucrat may decide I did not choose the appropriate "closest" code. And nothing is an error—it is always fraud. So, physicians are like rats in a maze where, no matter which way they turn, they get shocked. The Medicare reviewer three thousand miles away, who has never seen the patient and who has no medical training, decides you have mistakenly coded the procedure or "up-coded" (meaning chosen a higher level and more expensive code) the clinic visit, and Medicare denies your payment. Or worse, they see a "pattern" of up-coding and come after you with gun-toting federal agents to get big sums of money from you (the now-deemed "criminal" doctor) for overpayment and fines.

You may have heard that Medicare is broke. Well, one day, some Medicare guru looked around and found out where all the money went. Oh my! It went to doctors and hospitals. That presented a simple solution. When the famous bank robber Willy Sutton was asked, "Willy, why do you rob banks?" He answered, "Simple: that's where the money is!" Likewise, Medicare bureaucrats decided the simplest path to financial wellness was to go shake down doctors and hospitals. Since every doctor can be found to have committed coding/ billing errors, it is really just a matter of looking for easy assets and then bullying the physician into coughing up the dough. To do this, the government has turned to hired henchmen of the RAC (pronounced "rack") program. *RAC* stands for "recovery audit contractor," and the program makes me think of the Spanish Inquisition, or at least the Monty Python version of the Spanish Inquisition. The Pythons shout in their iconic skit, as they burst into an old lady's apartment unexpected, "No one expects the Spanish Inquisition!" And no physician expects his office to be raided and his staff and patients terrorized.

The RAC program is a civilian business, organized state by state, hired by the government for a percentage of the take. RACs aren't paid a dime by the government, but they receive 12 percent of all funds they collect from a medical provider. And they use the muscle of the government as the enforcer. If a staff member turns in a physician, that member can be rewarded with 10 percent of the reclaimed money. No doubt there is the occasional corrupt physician, but this is such a Robin Hood scheme rewarding the RAC and the "whistle-blowers" that considerable opportunity for corruption is apparent. (Keep this in mind when your longtime, seemingly honest physician is reported in your local newspaper as having committed Medicare fraud!)

Here's how it works. First, RACs find a physician with assets who may fall outside the bell curve on his choice of codes. The RAC reviewers make a case for up-coding, and call out the federal dogs. Federal agents then show up unannounced at the doctor's office (they don't need a warrant because, in the Orwellian world of government, even though you can be imprisoned as a result of the raid, technically, it isn't a "criminal" proceeding, just Medicare "compliance"). They may have guns drawn[2], may confiscate all your patient records (those that are not Medicare are taken so they can check for discrimination against Medicare patients), take your computers, and haul the doctor off in handcuffs.[3]

Then the extortion begins. The government plops down overwhelmingly large charges and tells the shaken physician that he or she owes enormous sums of money. Then they offer a deal. If the doctor will sign a privacy statement promising not to disclose what happened, the government will reduce the fines to a manageable sum. Of course, the government will publish in the news that the doctor has been found guilty of Medicare fraud and has been fined—that is a matter of public record—but the doctor can say nothing if he or she takes the deal. It is like what happened to Soviet citizens under the Cheka. When they were being hauled off in the middle of the night to the gulag or the Lubyanka, they were cautioned, "Go quietly, comrade; we don't want to disturb the neighbors."

Ninety-five percent of doctors roll over and sign. Five percent refuse, and the government then, to make them examples, often adds criminal charges to the civil ones. In fact, recently, Dr. John Natale, a highly competent and respected vascular surgeon for many years, was released from federal prison. He was not charged with murder, rape, money laundering, drug trafficking, or securities fraud. No, he sat in federal prison because a government prosecutor claimed he essentially mis-dictated an operative note.[4] At first, the Medicare squad tried to get him for overcharging the government. But he had the temerity to fight the charges in court, where it was shown he actually *undercharged* Medicare for his services. So having failed in easily squeezing his assets and having taken him to court, the Medicare squad created a new offense: they claimed he mis-dictated an operative report in an attempt to defraud the government. In the crazy world of Medicare, somehow having the wrong terms in an operative report (a fact disputed by several expert surgeons in this case) is enough to land you in jail. He spent ten months in federal penitentiary, and although I am not a lawyer, this seems to me to set a precedent not only in medicine but for nearly any business that does work for the government. Any form you fill out that is even remotely associated with billing can land you in jail for "fraud." As you can imagine, this risk of prosecution does not inspire physicians to live and work in areas filled with retirees where the physicians will be taking high volumes of Medicare and thus be subject to the whims of the Department of Justice.

Add to this the problems of central planning. As the Soviets discovered, central planning fails to anticipate market needs. The Central Committee could never predict how many tractors the farmers would need, so the Russian farmers either had too many (and not enough of some other machine) or too few, and the result was starvation. In modern medicine, ever since the 1970s the brainiacs in DC have used funding of medical education to regulate the number of doctors in the various specialties. I was in college in the late 1960s when students at liberal institutions of higher learning ran around sporting Mao jackets and waving the chairman's "Little Red Book." I suspect those are the very people in charge of deciding to cut the number of training slots for specialists, those holdovers from the sixties still being enamored of the concept of the "barefoot doctor." They have been preaching for years that we have too many specialists and need more primary care doctors. As a result, today we have only five thousand oncologists in the nation to treat our cancer patients. We have not added training seats in orthopaedics for many years in spite of increasing demand for total joint and trauma care. Nationwide, there are thirty thousand general surgeons, and twenty-four thousand orthopaedic surgeons. In the last twenty-five years, the number of general surgeons has declined 26 percent when compared to the population they serve. One-third of all surgeons are over fifty-five years old, and 30 percent say they would like to retire within the next several years. Yet we train only about 650 each year.[5] Ever tried to find a rheumatologist? Or a physiatrist (complex rehabilitation specialist)? They are rarer than hens' teeth. These doctor shortages are completely a result of the central planning of the 1970s.

Let's review what it takes to become a physician. Prior to 1960, many physicians became general practitioners (GPs). They had three to four years of college, four years of medical school, and a year of internship—seven to eight years in all. Today there are no GPs, and everyone does at least four years of college, four years of medical school, a year of internship, and two years of residency. A general, neurologic, or orthopaedic surgeon does four to six years of training after residency, so the total time to produce one surgeon from the time of graduation from high school is fourteen to sixteen years. As in industry, the longer the pipeline, the longer bad production decisions ripple through the economy.

In a free market, such shortages don't happen because the myriad observers and participants in the field make little day-to-day adaptations to increase or decrease production. But for years now, the hierarchy of graduate medical education has imposed Soviet-style central planning on the most precious commodity in medicine—the supply of physicians. Needless to say, predicting trends in populations as well as accounting for the rapidly changing science of medicine makes central planning of doctors impossible. But "central planners" keep trying. I have not found one specialty organization or one medical policy thinker who suggests letting demand for physicians determine the number of training positions available.

These shortages are about to get much worse: doctors are opting for early retirement or less productive shift work as hospital employees, and medical students are choosing specialties that have shorter training times and are not so damaging to their lifestyles. My son is a medical student at a private medical school. As he and his classmates discovered recently, they cannot pay back the cost of their medical education if they go into family practice or, in fact, anything but one of the top-paying specialties. And there are not enough training slots in the nation for everyone to do that.

I am an example of a highly trained physician being less productive than I would have been in a free market. I spent four years in college, four years in a private medical school, five years in orthopaedic residency, and a year of spine surgery fellowship. After all that, I worked for years in private practice. During those years, I worked eighty-plus-hour weeks, did six to twelve major spine cases a week, and took high-level orthopaedic trauma calls at a major regional medical center twice a week. I employed three full-time and four part-time employees. But one day I recognized I was on a treadmill running faster and faster just to pay my overhead. Ten years after being fully established in practice, having a three-month waiting list for my clinic visits, filling and overfilling my operative time every week, I was making less and less money, had less and less time for myself or my family, and became generally dissatisfied. Today, after twenty years in private practice, I work as a private contractor for a small community hospital in rural America. I work twenty hours a week, do no major spine surgery, and have no employees, but I fill a need in an underserved area. I have lots of free time to enjoy my friends and family, and I do nearly as well financially as I did before.

A word needs to be said here about the impact of income taxes on physicians. I am always amused when some politician says he or she is going to save small businesses by lowering the corporate income tax. Besides the fact that the tax lowering is usually in the few-percentage range, small businesses do not generally pay corporate taxes. They pass their profits through to their owners, who pay *personal income tax*. So to help, government must lower personal taxes. The personal income tax is especially damaging to physicians. Let's face it. Many other types of businesses are able to do some cash business or barter for goods and services—transactions that do not always make it to the 1040 report. On the other hand, doctors' incomes are almost exclusively from companies or the government, who faithfully report that income to the federal and state governments. We may be able to maximize the tax laws, but it is virtually impossible for us to hide income (and note to the IRS, having learned from Leona Helmsley, I would *never* try to do so). But on the gray and black fringes of the American economy, hiding income from the tax collector makes the difference between profitability and failure for many self-employed businesspeople.

In real terms, I am in the top tax bracket of 39.6 percent federal taxation. I pay 9 percent to the state, 8.5 percent in sales tax, and thousands in property taxes and local bonds. It is not an unreasonable estimate that more than 50 percent of my income goes to the government. Now, there are those who think doctors are rich and should belly up. Go ahead and keep thinking that, but at some point I am not going to work all night, standing in thirty-five pounds of lead, getting exposed to radiation and diseased blood and bone in order to give 50 percent of my labor to the government. I'd rather work less, have a life, and use my labor to my own ends—growing food, sewing clothing, building an add-on to my house, etc. And as more and more physicians have had the same epiphany, they, like me, have opted to work less. My podiatrist friend has an employed wife, also a professional. If she works more, he works less, since anything more would simply be taxed away. In Canada, a physician's pay is capped. If you do orthopaedic surgery or obstetrics, for example, after you have earned a certain amount, you can continue to see patients, but you will not get paid a dime more. Those physicians can be found in November and December in Florida, lounging on the beaches. In Sweden, an oncologist is paid for only a certain number of patients a day—then goes home early to fish. In America, we tax professionals into not working.

The government has made those doctors who are still working woefully inefficient by forcing them to comply with ever-more-complicated regulations—most notably by demanding they use electronic medical records (EMRs). Many physicians say they are at 50 percent productivity because of the electronic medical record. I know I am. What I can dictate in five minutes takes me twenty to forty minutes on the computer and still results in an inferior note. When I dictated my notes, I could see twenty or more patients in the morning and have my dictations mostly done. Now, I see fewer patients and save all charting till after work, thus lengthening my day for no financial benefit and to the detriment of accurate patient history.

In sum, in the near future, as doctor retirements accelerate, there will be many underserved areas. Finding a doctor will be harder and harder, especially for the poor, the rural, and the elderly. In chapter 14, I discuss the strategies for finding a doctor who will be there when you need him or her, and for alternatives to the classic MD or DO.

Finally, the government has so overregulated medical education that the young doctors today are not trained to the former high standards. I know this firsthand having watched my son go through four years of medical school. When I went through medical school, I delivered thirty-four babies. He has delivered zero. When I trained I was always starting IVs and drawing blood. If he had not worked with me at my hospital, he would not know how to start an IV, and he is a senior medical student! Between fears of liability and the Medicare regulations, students today do not get their hands dirty, figuratively speaking, of course. Years ago Libby Zion was a patient at a teaching hospital in New York who died of cardiac arrest. Her lawyer father sued claiming it was due to poor judgment by the student residents because of their long shifts at the hospital. After that the government decided students and residents should be limited in the hours they can be in the hospital working. Now if residents are in the middle of a surgery case when their hours are up, they must scrub out and leave it to others—a luxury not afforded to surgeons in private practice. During my surgical residency we joked that the problem with being on call only every other night was that you missed 50 percent of the good cases. Today's residents are taught a blue-collar shift work mentality, which has no place in the care of patients or the practice of medicine. And they are not getting trained. The advisor for my son's surgical candidates has told them they should plan on doing another year of training after the five-year general surgery residency because those five years will not give them enough training to be competent! So when we look at physician man-hours in America, we must understand that a newly minted physician will be able to handle less than those trained in previous decades.

3

WHY YOUR DOCTOR IS OUT OF DATE

n 1976, during medical school, I listened while the lecturer in biochemistry explained why the optimum dose of aspirin to prevent clotting in heart vessels was 82 milligrams, or one baby aspirin a day, not the two-aspirin-a-day regimen used at that time. Yet in 1996, when I was first in practice in Arizona, I noticed that most patients were still taking two full aspirin for this purpose—a dose shown over twenty years before to actually work *against* the desired effect by turning off the anticlotting mechanism of the arterial wall.

I was shocked to think that doctors were practicing twenty-year-old medicine, employing a regimen that was in direct conflict with basic biochemistry. Subsequently I have learned this is not the exception but is the abysmal mode of practice in America. There are at least three major factors that have contributed to this sad state of affairs: state medical boards, clinical "groupthink," and an ineffective approach to information gathering. (Additionally, some doctors are wrong in their approach—not necessarily out of date, but just flat-out wrong—due to drug company propaganda.)

In any aspect of life, there have always been the herd and those who break out of the herd with new ideas. Galileo broke from the pack to change our view of the solar system; George Eastman threw out wet plates in favor of dry photo plates and overnight changed photography. Joseph Lister revolutionized surgery with carbolic acid antisepsis. These people became leaders by adopting different perspectives on old problems. But if Joseph Lister were alive today and proposed carbolic acid for asepsis, he would risk being sanctioned, even de-licensed, by his state medical board. Why? Because state medical boards use the concept of "standard of care" in determining if a physician is right or wrong in his or her treatment. If you are practicing the methods used by 90 percent of your peers, you are "correct," but if your treatment falls within that other 10 percent, you are *wrong by definition.* Never mind that within that 10 percent are the new, improved ideas in any specialty. This concept of "standard of care" is an absolutely guaranteed formula for mediocrity that would ruin any other industry. Imagine if the electronic industry used this method for evaluating good engineering design. We would be using rotary phones and an abacus! Edison and Tesla would have been jailed in such a society. Yet we accept this worldview as normal in medicine. As I am writing this, the number one reason for being taken to task by a state medical board (punishment can range from a letter of reprimand to taking away a doctor's medical license) is "overtreatment" of hypothyroidism. Unfortunately, medical boards are using outdated science to punish up-to-date physicians.

Hypothyroidism is a common condition—some estimate 80 percent of Americans suffer some degree of this abnormality. In hypothyroidism, the gland in the neck that produces thyroid hormone fails to produce enough to run the body's systems. Thyroid hormones are like the fuel for your metabolic furnace. Inside every cell in the body are little mitochondria, which are the power generators of the cells. Thyroid hormones control the activity of the mitochondria as your thermostat controls your furnace. Too much of the hormones and your body temperature is set higher, your metabolism goes up, and you can experience a variety of problems, such as heart fluttering, anxiety, and unwanted weight loss. "Low thyroid" means your thyroid doesn't produce enough hormones, and the opposite happens: your body shuts down the furnace (mitochondria) so your temperature goes down and metabolic processes are slowed. This results in always feeling cold—cold hands and feet—loss of eyebrows and eyelashes, weight gain, depression and slow thinking, sluggishness, thyroid nodules, an enlarged thyroid gland, or diminished heart function. To work well, the thyroid has to have several things—stimulation from TSH or "thyroid-stimulating hormone," iodine as a basic building block of the hormone, and selenium for the enzyme system that makes the hormone active. Hypothyroidism happens when any or all of these are deficient.

The American diet is woefully deficient in iodine. Iodine has many good properties, including an anticancer effect, but mostly it is necessary to produce thyroid hormone. The Midwest, where I live, has been known as the "goiter belt" because our diet traditionally had little seafood and, thus, little iodine. Iodine used to be added to food as a stabilizer, but unfortunately, after World War II, bromine was substituted for iodine. This is bad for several reasons. First, bromine is not iodine, so it doesn't help make thyroid hormone. Second, bromine inhibits the uptake of iodine from the gut, thereby lowering your ability to absorb the iodine from your food. And finally, bromine is taken into cells, where it mimics iodine and again inhibits its function. (In the next section, on wellness, I emphasize a wheat-free diet as a formula for avoiding doctors, but if you do eat wheat, avoid the "brominated" variety. You will see some flour advertised as "never bleached, never brominated." Iodized salt gives you very little of the daily requirement. In chapter 11, I discuss how to supplement your iodine correctly.)

Then there are genetic drift factors, disease, medications, bad diet, and other things that produce hypothyroidism, making it one of the most common disorders, if not the most common, that we see (or ignore) in medicine. The classic test for hypothyroidism is checking the thyroid-stimulating hormone (TSH) levels, which go up as the thyroid fails. The body makes more and more TSH to try to flog the thyroid gland into doing its thing. Traditionally, the normal range of TSH is based on an "average" level in the population and was thought to be 0.4 to 2.5 (recently lowered from 5.5). But basic science shows that your metabolism and, specifically, your cardiac output (the ability of your heart muscle to pump blood) is not optimum until your TSH is under 1.0. I never thought of myself as being hypothyroid, but having heard a lecture on this subject, I tested my own TSH and found it to be 1.9. Now, using "standard" medical care, this would not be treated. But using the new scientific understanding, I started myself on low-dose thyroid (I had already been taking an iodine supplement). Amazingly, within months my hands and feet warmed up, I regrew my eyelashes, which I thought were just sparse due to age, and my eyebrows filled out. I lost about five pounds and had more exercise tolerance.

But here is the catch. Medical boards are prosecuting doctors for using such knowledge and experience in treating their patients. A general surgery friend of mine gave up surgery practice later in life to do "anti-aging medicine." Having heard of the actions of medical boards, he approached the Medical Board of California proactively and asked about their approach to treating hypothyroidism. Specifically he asked if it were true that overtreatment was the most common reason for sanctioning doctors. They confirmed that it was. Then he asked them what were their criteria for sanctioning doctors. The police officer on the board—not a physician, the police officer!—responded, "a TSH under 2.5." My surgeon friend decided to practice in another state, but you see the point. It is not science driving how you are treated by your doctor, but fear of—dare I say, totalitarian—medical boards.

Few things in life are as powerful as peer pressure. Physicians—like football players, stockbrokers, and many others—tend to slap each other on the back (at least figuratively) and aspire to be in the "in crowd." They reinforce mainstream beliefs at professional meetings and in publications while ignoring the unpopular guys—even though the ideas of the unpopular guys may ultimately prove correct. Famous examples include the ridicule given the proposals that stomach ulcers come from bacteria, that viruses can cause cancer, that germs cause disease—all of which were proven true. Publication in medical journals, while supposedly peer-reviewed without knowledge of the author, tends to favor those with connections to the reviewers, or at least papers reinforcing the reviewers' views. I once tried to publish the result of performing a new surgical technique, which I had used successfully in more than seventy patients, only to be told in the written denial, "Everyone knows you can't do that." (The technique is now in fairly widespread use.)

Physicians and researchers holding contrarian views may be ostracized, criticized, and actually humiliated. Take, for example, Warren S. Warren, who was rudely roasted at Princeton and whose funding was threatened. Ultimately, his finding of anomalous MRI interactions was proven correct, resulting in improved MRI technology. But not before he faced mockery from his peers.

Recently, Andrew Wakefield, a formerly university-based British gastroenterologist, published a case report series concerning possible side effects of the MMR vaccine. As a result, he has had his reputation impugned, his medical license revoked, and his book censored from publication in Britain. Of course, a case report is only supposed to describe a clinician's observations, thereby giving others a chance to either confirm the findings or refute them. But Wakefield has been charged with "falsification of data" (a charge he has reliably refuted in court), intent to defraud, and malpractice. Why? Because he made an observation outside the groupthink belief that *all vaccines are safe in all children.* In this case, the groupthink is reinforced by government self-protection and big pharmaceutical company money. (It goes without much saying that government research funding is not generally given to the minority opinion, so again, the same ideas are reinforced.) Whatever the truth is, history tends to uphold the beliefs of those whose writings were censored, not the agencies doing the censoring. In cases such as Dr. Wakefield's, the abusive treatment of the physician—simply for reporting his observations—has had a chilling effect on those who might come forward with supportive data. Once again, physicians are afraid to advance real knowledge if it does not conform to the accepted norm. And you, the patient/customer, are given yesterday's medical information.

Adding insult to injury is the creeping odium of consensus in science—the notion that truth is discovered by majority vote among investigators, not by careful application of testing and scientific method. As Michael Crichton—a physician as well as an author—said in 2003, in a speech at Cal Tech:

> Let's be clear: the work of science has nothing whatever to do with consensus. Consensus is the business of politics. Science, on the contrary, requires only one investigator who happens to be right, which means that he or she has results that are verifiable by reference to the real world. In science consensus is irrelevant. What are relevant are reproducible results. The greatest scientists in history are great precisely because they broke with the consensus. There is no such thing as consensus science. If it's consensus, it isn't science. If it's science, it isn't consensus. Period.[1]

"Best practice," is the new idea for improving medicine through standardization. It is essentially consensus applied to medicine. University clinicians decide on the best way to treat something; then this is written down in an algorithmic form and disseminated to all doctors. For example, we are told that it is best practice to give antibiotics within forty-five minutes of the surgical incision. So all over the country, hospitals attempt to comply by giving the antibiotic within forty-five minutes of the start of all operations. Predictably, what was first sold as a suggestion now is becoming law, reinforced by government and insurance third-party payers: fail to follow best practice and we will fail to pay you. So now, Medicare penalizes hospitals if the antibiotic is given forty-six minutes before cut time, instead of the maximum of forty-five.

Unfortunately such clinical dogma ignores the fact that people are individuals with individualized problems. While the algorithmic approach may apply 90 percent of the time and may be a useful learning tool or reference point, the good physician needs to be able to vary treatment when his patient's problem varies from the norm. In orthopaedics, for example, we are told to "anticoagulate all hip fracture patients" (give blood thinners) because, statistically, patients with hip fractures are at risk of dangerous blood clotting in their legs. But if the patient's fracture is fixed in a minimally invasive way within hours of the trauma and the patient mobilized the same day, does he or she really need Lovenox or Coumadin, with its attendant risks? Do we thin our blood with chemicals every time we go to sleep? Of course not, and to treat these patients with blood thinner increases their risks for bleeding and hemorrhagic stroke while, at the same time, not really making a difference in their risk of clinically important blood clots. In other words, it adds risk without benefit—a classic formula for bad medical care. Uniformity of thought leads to mediocrity of science and inappropriateness of care.

Evidence-based medicine (EBM)—the latest government/university brainchild—only makes this problem worse. It sounds good. Evidence. What's not to like? But EBM is an upside-down approach to medical progress. In the past, clinicians faced with a new or unusual medical problem were allowed to think. They were able to offer treatment they thought might be effective as long as the treatment would "first do no harm." Patient safety always came first. They based their treatment decisions not only on the literature but also on their understanding of basic science, their clinical experience, and their judgment. With EBM, on the other hand, we doctors are *prohibited* from offering treatment unless we can show, preferably with "high-powered" long-term studies, that the treatment is effective. In other words, I might think this new treatment will work for your unique problem, but I have to prove through long-term studies (often taking decades) that my idea actually works *before* I can use it on you, the sick patient. Of course, you will be dead or crippled before this can be done.

A clinician with good common sense and good ideas cannot act without a paper trail backup of some published study. In spite of the acknowledged inadequacies (and actual falsification at times) of the medical literature, all emphasis is placed on these studies, and no credit is given to clinical skill. This has led to incredible statistical gymnastics being applied to collections of studies generating meta-analysis papers that resemble numerology more than clinical medicine. And of course anything that is not a double blind study is questioned. A double blind study is one in which two groups of people are studied—one group is given the real drug, the other group a placebo having no clinical effect (sugar tablet, for example). And it is double-blind because neither the investigator nor the patients know ahead of time who is getting the real or false drug. Now, this makes sense for some things, such as pain medication or diabetic drugs, but not to everything we do in medicine. But when government gets a new hammer, everything starts looking like a nail, and government bureaucrats seldom have the scientific understanding to curdle milk, let alone decide on the effectiveness of complex reconstructive surgical procedures.

Recently some British wags published a parody on this approach, entitled, "Parachute use to prevent death and major trauma related to gravitational challenge: systematic review of randomized controlled trials."[2] Their point was that we use parachutes although no powerful double-blind study exists to prove that they work. They recommended at the end that those academicians raising such a ruckus about EBM be the first to volunteer as testers to see if parachutes really make a difference. Of course, if such a study were to be done, the EBM promoter "volunteers" would be pushed (I doubt they would jump) out of a perfectly good aircraft, and neither they nor the study investigator could know ahead of time whether their parachute bags *actually* contained parachutes or if they were "placebos." As they point out, tongue-in-British-cheek but quite convincingly, EBM really does not apply to everything. Some things, such as appendectomies and using a parachute, are just commonsense to do. When considering evidence-based medicine, I am reminded of James Thurber's quote, "You might as well fall flat on your face as to lean too far over backwards."

Finally, how do we learn new things? It was said of Sir Isaac Newton that, when at Cambridge, he had learned all the science there was to know at the time. Today, it is difficult to stay abreast of even a small portion of available knowledge. And we are particularly ill equipped in medicine to make best use of the knowledge at hand since we approach medical learning much like the processional caterpillar. The processional caterpillar is named because of its habit of following a leader. No one knows how the leader is chosen, but before slithering to or from feeding grounds, the unchosen caterpillars form a line behind the leader. If, however, such caterpillars are placed on the rim of a bucket, the leader will eventually catch up to the end of the line, conclude he has been replaced, and start to follow the caterpillar in front of him until they are all going around and around the bucket rim, following each other over the same ground again and again. What a metaphor for medical education! Residents learn from outdated texts and outdated staff and each other; then they teach interns and medical students, who then become residents; and the knowledge is passed around like the caterpillars on the bucket rim. In 1976, while the biochemists were teaching us that one baby aspirin was optimal, generations of senior residents were teaching interns that they should prescribe two full aspirins—the lesson they had in turn been taught by their senior residents—and it would take years before level one studies would appear to countermand that dictum.

Additionally, earlier and more rigid subspecialization has stovepiped learning into narrower and narrower brackets. Specialists may solve a problem in their own realm without realizing the problems their treatments have created in another specialist's area of expertise. The classic example of this is the use of "statin" drugs to lower serum cholesterol. Although statins have not been shown to decrease all-cause mortality from heart disease, they are being prescribed to more and more patients. As the drug companies with government backing produce more of these "guidelines" for use of statins, more and more adults will qualify for a statin prescription. Unfortunately, the cardiologist who prescribes the statin may see the patient's chest pain improve, but that doctor won't realize that the patient's worsening dementia is due to the drastic lowering of cholesterol needed for brain function, because as the patient's memory deteriorates, he doesn't see the cardiologist; he sees a neurologist. Or when the patient gets muscle cramping and pain, he sees the orthopaedist, and when he gets diabetes, he sees his primary care doc or an endocrinologist. So the cardiologist prescribes statins, blissfully unaware of the actual impact on other body systems. And this is just one drug example, but there are many others. To make this problem worse, as fewer physicians see their own patients in the hospitals (because of the use of hospitalists to cover inpatients) there is less and less face-to-face interaction between doctors of different disciplines—perhaps the best arena for cross-pollination of ideas.

I have often quipped that we need a Journal of Good Ideas—a non-peer-reviewed publication where physicians can report their experiences and ideas that might prove helpful to others, without the need for high-powered proof before publication. For example, it has been my observation that many problems in postoperative inpatients can be averted by ensuring that their caffeine levels are maintained. I have neither the time nor the resources to do the kind of study required to prove this in a standard medical journal, but it is a simple observation that can be tried by others. (Trust me—less time for bowel recovery, fewer headaches, less fatigue, and better postoperative mobilization!)

Fortunately, a new forum for truly out-of-the-box thinking has arisen. The fastest-growing subset of medicine today is in the field of "anti-aging." The title may be a misnomer, but this area of medical research and practice is dedicated to optimizing health throughout an extended life span. In their journals and their meetings, anti-aging physicians of all specialties and interests discuss improving health, utilizing not *only* the published long-term literature but also their experience and understanding of *basic science*—in short, they have gone back to the way it once was. The anti-aging medical leaders scour the medical literature *across all disciplines* for ideas and evidence. Then, instead of erecting barriers for the sharing of knowledge, they publish ideas with extensive documentation in non-peer-reviewed magazines and let the discerning physician reach conclusions about the validity of the ideas presented. In essence, they have become the Google search engine for medical information and have combined that knowledge in unique and useful ways.

State medical boards, peer review, best practices, and evidence-based medicine are put forth to improve the quality of medicine and promote safety for the patient. But how many patients die or are disabled due to lost opportunity, inability for ideas to be promulgated, and physicians' fear of being sanctioned for providing the avant-garde, not just the standard care?

You, the patient, should understand where your doctor is "coming from" as the jargon goes. If your doctor is the classic medical school graduate, she is probably a member of this "Flat Earth Society" (as I once was) that buys into the EBM and best practices and the board regimens. Not to say she is a bad doctor, just that she sees the world in a very stylized fashion. She does not recognize the limitations of the medical literature, the inability of current laboratory tests to really assess deficient states, and the straitjacket of treatment options imposed by the "authorities."

I would opt for a doctor with a standard degree of MD or DO who advertises "complementary" and/or "integrative" or "anti-aging" medicine. These doctors can be found in yellow pages and via world-health.net, or through the Cenegenics organization, among other sources. As an added benefit, these docs often work for cash, so they will be the "last ones standing" when Medicare crashes and burns. Sometimes it is just word of mouth, but today there are very few cities without such physicians, and it is worth seeking true preventive care from them.

4

THE FINAL GOVERNMENT TAKEOVER

As the current medical system collapses of its own internal inconsistencies, people who have been conditioned to look to government for solutions will predictably look to the federal government for help. And government being government will never ignore the chance of using a crisis to further its agenda of power and growth.

But let's look around us. How has government done in the fields of education, banking, the post office, or the DMV?

In Iowa, in the old days, before the Department of Education was created, every small town of three hundred people or more could afford its own school building and teachers. The local school officials provided order and discipline, and the local elected school board controlled the curriculum. Iowa had one of the highest literacy rates and best academic record in the nation, and it became famous for its Iowa Test of Basic Skills. But now, in spite of spending nearly twelve thousand dollars per student, the twenty-fourth highest spending per pupil in the nation, Iowa ranks thirty-fifth on the ACT in composite scores and forty-first in science. Children who once were able to walk to school (and we wonder about obesity?) are bused or driven to distant conglomerate schoolhouses, while the grand old buildings of yesteryear molder and decay. We have no local control over curriculum, and little to say about teacher hiring and firing.

Around the turn of the last century, my grandfather and father both were educated in one-room schoolhouses with children of all ages. Both were well-educated men, literate, with Palmer penmanship and math skills. My grandfather "graduated" with an eighth grade education, but my father went on to three doctorate degrees and a teaching stint at Harvard in biochemistry. From a dingy little one-room schoolhouse to an old, no-frills, brick high school in a town of one thousand souls, to Harvard. No state or federal tax dollars involved. Just a lot of honest hard work and straight thinking.

Today, with tax dollars spent at every level, at $12,000 per pupil, a class of twenty-five students could afford paying a teacher $150,000 per year, rent of $60,000 per year, and contribute $50,000 toward the salaries of a principal and secretary (that's all the administrators I had when I graduated in 1969 from high school), and still have $90,000 a year left over for books and incidentals.

Now, I know this is a bit oversimplified, but small businesses would look at it this way. Before drilling down to line items, they would get a big-picture view of where the money is spent. In our administration-heavy education system, where does the money go? Well, simple. It goes to government-ponderous bureaucracy. According to its own website, the US Department of Education in 2010 had nearly forty-three hundred employees and a budget of $60 billion. And they don't actually teach one child. The Iowa Department of Education spent more than $6.5 million on administration of a total budget of $7 billion, which included such non-school-related items as Iowa Public Television, family support and parental education, special ed services from birth to age three, the state library, and the Entrepreneurs with Disabilities Program. In sum, when government gets involved, money is taken from the direct consumer, and instead of going directly to the producer—i.e., teachers and schools—it is siphoned away into murky, back-hall budgets made for the benefit of other interests—the support of outdated book depositories, social workers produced in excess of market need, and programs perpetuating nonessential jobs for government employees. And now we are forced into Common Core—a plan so bad that even unionized teachers are balking. It promises to double the rate of student testing, at a cost of thirty dollars per student per test, and requires all new textbooks—money that goes to the private corporations and consortia that hold the copyright. And it has no proven benefit—quite the opposite. It says something when federal agents are being placed into classrooms to ensure compliance to the "Common Core" standards.[1]

Every small town has had its own bank, and usually more than one, but a small bank's ability to exist independently is in jeopardy due to government involvement. The gross overregulation disproportionately hurts the small bank. Bank examiners used to show up every two to three years, but now there are examiners from various agencies twice or more a year, and the banks pay the cost of their own audits. Before the Federal Reserve was established in 1913, banks of all sizes and types were truly private and independent, and although in those days some failed (taking their clients with them), relatively few people were affected. Before government intervention in banking, we never had prolonged national boom-and-bust cycles with systemic toxicity (e.g., the recent real estate debacle or the Bear-Stearns collapse or, indeed, the Great Depression).

For those who think the Federal Reserve is only an insurance device for banks, the so-called FDIC guarantee, think again. As Thomas DiLorenzo points out, the Fed is responsible for regulating

> bank holding companies, state-chartered banks, foreign branches of member banks, edge and agreement corporations, state-licensed branches, agencies, and representative offices of foreign banks, nonbanking activities of foreign banks, national banks, savings banks, nonbank subsidiaries of bank holding companies, financial reporting procedures, accounting policies of banks, business "continuity" in case of economic emergencies, consumer protection laws, securities dealings of banks,

information technology used by banks, foreign investment by banks, foreign lending by banks, branch banking, bank mergers and acquisitions, who may own a bank, capital "adequacy standards," extensions of credit for the purchase of securities, equal opportunity lending, mortgage disclosure information, reserve requirements, electronic funds transfers, interbank liabilities, Community Reinvestment Act subprime lending demands, all international banking operations, consumer leasing, privacy of consumer financial information, payments on demand deposits, "fair credit" reporting, transactions between member banks and their affiliates, truth in lending, and truth in savings.[2]

The issues of federal government involvement in banking are complicated, but the effects are very obvious once you know what you are looking at. Whereas interest rates were once based on real market forces, now the "Fed" sets the rates to suit its own and the administration's goals. This has led to outrageously low interest rates, which may be good for the first-time home owner, but anyone living on interest from bonds or savings is being devastated by the nearly zero interest rates set by the Federal Reserve Bank.

Small banks that cannot afford navigating the regulatory morass are closing or being purchased by larger and larger conglomerates. We are left with fewer banks, less competition, and ultimately a less safe, less customer-friendly banking environment.

Banks have become the action arm of the government's social policies. Fannie Mae and Freddie Mac, at the heart of the 2008–09 financial implosion, were specifically told by several administrations to lower requirements for home-buying to allow more lower-income families to buy homes. Under Eric Holder, the Department of Justice has doubled down on this failed policy, ordering banks such as Midwest BankCentre to provide "special financing" in the predominantly black areas of St. Louis for conventional home loan financing at a fixed prime rate for borrowers "who would ordinarily not qualify for such rates for reasons including the lack of required credit quality, income or down payment."[3]

Then of course, there are the post office and the DMV. Given that your time has any value at all, why would you ever choose either of these over the private alternatives, FedEx and UPS pickup and delivery? They travel the world. They are fast and reliable. No standing in long lines in a post office. How nice is it to get your first motor vehicle license through a private dealer rather than your DMV or other similar government-licensing bureau?

Government may supply jobs to the chosen, but government—any government at any level—produces *nothing*, including medical care. The only way government can possibly supply medical care is to forcibly requisition the components from the private sector—what is left of it at the time. Doctors will be forced into government servitude. Hospitals will be nationalized. Patients will be given their national health service identification, and we will all be locked into the type of system that has failed around the world.

"Obamacare," or PPACA (the "Patient Protection and Affordable Care Act)," was passed over the objections of the great majority of Americans. The system it installs is perfectly designed to destroy private medicine and bring about single-party payer, Canadian-style, universal health care. There are two points worth discussing for the purposes of predicting the future and understanding the present—the role of HHS (the Department of Health and Human Services) and the design of these "accountable care organizations" (ACOs).

Congresswoman Nancy Pelosi famously said that the Congress and Senate needed to pass Obamacare so everyone would know what was in the bill. As outrageous as that statement sounds concerning the nature of our elected officials, the truth is even uglier. In fact, it doesn't matter what is in the bill—and never did. The twenty-four hundred pages of Obamacare could be an untranslated Greek ode—it would make no difference.[4] The only thing of importance is the one line in the bill that authorizes the Department of Health and Human Services (HHS) to write regulations for implementing Obamacare—*regulations that carry the force of law.*

According to the US Constitution, the only body of people

that can write laws is the United States Congress. But Congress has abrogated this constitutional responsibility and has allowed unelected bureaucrats to write millions of pages of regulations that can land you in prison or fine away your life's savings. Only a few months into Obamacare its 2,400 pages were already dwarfed by the pages of regulations being spewed out at a rate unfathomable to the normal nonbureaucratic human mind. Now, this is not unique to HHS. EPA, Treasury, Agriculture, and other departments put vast ink to vast paper, but the leaders, by orders of magnitude, in pumping out economically damaging regulations, are HHS toadies. In 2011 five departments—Treasury, Commerce, Agriculture, Interior, and EPA—won the prize for prolific regulation writing by collectively pumping out 1,733 regulations.[5] In fact in 2014, the Competitive Enterprise Institute's annual survey of the federal regulatory state, *Ten Thousand Commandments,* estimated the total federal regulatory burden at $1.8 trillion per year. The tax burden Americans face is less than the regulatory burdens imposed on them.

But if you look specifically at the number of regulations that have more than $100 million impact on our economy, the Department of Health and Human Services is in the lead all by itself. Sixty-five regulations with more than a $100 million impact on the economy were in the pipeline of HHS by the close of 2011. The next closest contender was the Environmental Protection Agency, with only twenty-one regulations. And I used to think the EPA was pretty damaging.

Keep in mind that this nation once existed with only eleven written pages of law—the Constitution if typewritten today. Now we have more than fifty-four feet of the Federal Register used to imprison and enslave us. (We have nine pages just on the disposal of the newly mandated curlicue lightbulbs!) We have people in jail for unwittingly importing the wrong subspecies of crustacean or for choosing the wrong CPT code for billing a medical procedure.

The upshot of all this regulation is that medicine has become like a very inefficient machine, spewing out heat but not moving anything forward. We spend so much time in "compliance" with regulations that little actual medical care can get done. Look around at the hospitals. There are fewer patient care areas and vastly more administrative suites. And God help the private practitioner who does not have the large workforce to navigate the regulatory stream.

Now enter ACOs—accountable care organizations. If I were intending to create collapse of the free market health system, I could do no better than in implementing ACOs. As I write this, ACOs are being created all over the country. Today ACOs are "virtual" patient care areas centered on a regional medical center or large urban hospital. In phase one, a bureaucrat negotiates with a hospital center and gives it an ACO designation. He goes to a map and draws a circle around the hospital to create a patient catchment area for which the new hospital/ACO is responsible. At first these ACOs are "virtual," meaning that patients can get care wherever they want, but if they fall into a particular circle, they become simply a statistic for that ACO.

To better understand how this plays out, let's take a prototype patient, Jane Doe. Mrs. Doe is a widow living on the family farm in Guthrie County, Iowa. The nearest hospital is in the town of Guthrie Center, but her doctor is in Panora, which is closer to her home. She is now a member of the Guthrie County Hospital ACO centered at the hospital in Guthrie Center. She signed no papers, is not yet aware of any change in her health care options because she receives Medicare benefits, and is still with her long-term doctor. She has no knowledge of being a member of the ACO, because it is "virtual," like a computer game, and she is represented by an avatar who is just an ACO statistic at this point.

Unlike a computer game, though, this has real-world consequences, because now, the "virtual" ACO begins to send volumes of data about its patients—including Jane Doe—to the federal government. This information includes every bill generated on every patient—whether they are government or private pay. It includes the most private medical information. Mrs. Doe's history of depression is now in the hands of a government bureaucrat, as is her history of pregnancies, abortions, her past smoking history, and her weight and height—her body mass index. The government compares the cost of her care through the ACO to the cost of the same care outside the ACO. If the ACO care is cheaper, the ACO is rewarded with bonus money equal to one-half of the so-called cost savings.

So Mrs. Doe sees her private non-ACO doctor for wrist pain. He knows the biggest issue is really depression and loneliness, so he spends some time with her to talk about her life and coping with being recently widowed. For this he charges a certain CPT code based on the extra time he spent and the diagnoses. This price is then compared to the cost of seeing an ACO physician in the multiphysician complex. Those physicians may or may not have long-term relationships with their patients, so they may or may not be as sensitive to her as a whole person. It is my experience in big, government-funded groups that patients are treated generically, not as individuals, and shuttled from doctor to doctor. (Think the Veteran Affairs or Indian Health Service where doctors come and go every few years.) And it is my experience that private care is generally cheaper than big organizational care, but in this scenario, the ACOs will have the advantage of reporting. They will mobilize countless minions to massage the data so the ACOs look good to the government and garner the money prize. (We just saw this happen in the recent VA scandal where the numbers were massaged to improve bonuses for the administrators.) Just the reporting alone will drive many private docs to give up and join the ACOs.

The ACO statisticians in the federal government will also compare apples to oranges. Whereas the private doc will charge for the time he spent with the patient—and it was time well spent but not really about her wrist—at the ACO, such a patient will be seen briefly only about the wrist, so the cost will be cheaper, but the care will be more superficial.

The upshot of all this is that the private doctors will be "shown" to be more costly and will not be the ones favored to win the bonus money. Notice that even if the private guys give cheaper care, they reap no monetary reward—only the ACOs get a bonus for cost-effectiveness and no penalty for the times they exceed private cost. So who will win? Predictably, private practice will be squeezed out of existence. It is already now scarcer and scarcer to find young people going into truly private practice. And according to a 2012 physician survey, only 48.5 percent of physicians are in private practice, but private practice was nearly universal before the advent of Medicare and Medicaid. And the decrease in numbers of private practitioners is a fact agreed upon by all parties looking at the ACO effect.[6] (The issue is whether one believes this to be good or bad and whether one believes this is a conscious effort of the ACO push.)

During phase two, the government will harden these ACOs into *real* catchment areas, and patients—at least those enrolled in Obamacare, Medicare, and other federal programs—will not have a choice of mobility. They will have to stay with a particular ACO. At this point, Mrs. Doe now knows she is a member of an ACO. She has been registered and been given identification data. She will be told who her primary care doctor is (or physician's assistant or nurse practitioner. Since there are already insufficient physicians to go around, those in practice are working fewer hours on average and seeing fewer patients than four years ago, and 62 percent are planning on early retirement[7]). Mrs. Doe may be unhappy at losing her longtime doc, and she probably doesn't like driving farther to the new conglomerate ACO hospital complex. But while she is unhappy, the ACO administrators will be rejoicing at all the bonus money they are now receiving and the proverbial "pats on the head" they are getting from their masters at HHS for being "the chosen" to practice great, cost-effective medicine. These ACO fat cats are naive at best, corrupt at worst, because the government never leaves free money on the table and because the goal is not to make ACOs succeed but to make them the "fall guy."

With phase three, the sucker punch hits. When the last remnants of private practice are driven out of existence, there will be no "cost savings," as there will be no one left for the ACOs to be compared to. America will have been totally divided up into these government-funded ACOs, and, as the money is generally withdrawn, they will all start to fail—virtually simultaneously, from smallest to largest systems. Under a free market, or even Medicare, hospitals individually would sometimes fail. But others would prosper. In the third phase of the ACO collapse, however, the government, by ensnaring everyone into the same economic quagmire, will have staged a great orchestrated collapse. And just like the Reichstag fire—a crisis perpetrated by the Nazis so they could supply their own totalitarian solution—this crisis will be the excuse for more government. As hospitals all over the nation become financially distressed and medical care delivery begins to fall apart, the government will call for *single-party payer universal health care* to save the day. (Of course this single party Canadian plan was the goal all along.)

What is happening now to our Mrs. Jane Doe? Well, at first her appointment times were a little delayed, but now she may wait months for routine appointments. Her small hospital system failed and has been consolidated into the closest large system, but this now means a drive of more than sixty miles. For her routine care she usually sees a PA or nurse practitioner, no longer a physician, and even then sees a different one nearly every visit. Her records are all on the computerized system, and her data have long been in the hands of Washington paper pushers. These "reviewers" have run computer scans on records to look for outliers and have determined that she is receiving care that is not warranted at her age of seventy-two. She will be taken off her Coumadin for atrial fibrillation (a heart rhythm disorder) and just given an aspirin a day, since her "disability-adjusted life-year" cost benefit analysis shows that a stroke would not cause too many productive life years lost (as it would if she were thirty-five).[8] And the same nonmedical bureaucrats are denying her cardiologist's request for a pacemaker to solve the atrial fibrillation problem—for the same reason: she is just too damn old to warrant such expenditure of government funds. (This is already happening under Medicare but will ramp up in the new world medical order.)

And you will know, when you see the collapse of more and more small hospital centers, that the end is near—not just the end of high-quality medical care but the end of America as we know it. We will be breathing our last gasps of liberty. Because if the government controls your very health, what will it not take from you—mostly in the name of "safety"?

Needless to say, there will be pockets of resistance—doctors who quit and doctors who will continue to operate for cash. Since the cash practices will be more caring, patient centered, and will provide real medicine, they will have to be eradicated so the public will not see the contrast. Doctors will most likely face prosecution if they attempt to take payment for services rendered. This has happened elsewhere. For years, it has been illegal in Canada, North Korea, and Cuba for physicians to take direct payment from their patients. Currently, since Canada is actually allowing some cash pay and Cuba has renounced total communism, there is only one country that totally criminalizes private medicine—North Korea. But we are working on it. The state of Vermont has voted in a single-party payer system, and it remains to be seen if they will actually prosecute those doctors who choose to opt out. If they do, they will be in fine company—North Korea and Vermont—what a pair.

A black market of sorts will no doubt develop, as it did in the Soviet Union. One former Soviet citizen's husband recalled to me how his wife's uncle got his gall bladder surgery. Although Soviet health care was free and universal, it was like commodities in the GUM, the state-controlled department store—nonexistent. When the uncle became desperately ill, the family saved up anything they could buy—shoes, food, household goods, and so forth, and bribed the surgeon and the anesthesiologist. That former Soviet citizen recalled to me how the doctors "borrowed" equipment from a local hospital, took it to the family's tiny apartment, and removed the diseased gall bladder on the family's kitchen table—probably a cleaner spot than the hospital operating room.

Single-source medical care is lousy. The longer such a system exists, the worse it becomes. By the time the Berlin Wall fell and we could peek into the world of Soviet medicine, for example, 57 percent of Soviet hospitals had no hot water, and 36 percent had no running water at all. There were dead cats lying in the hallways, and a legion of babies were exposed to HIV because needles were reused without sterilization. While the free market was advancing to MRIs and sophisticated robotic surgery, the Soviets, with vast natural resources, were descending into a level of medicine about on par with the czarist era. And this system was created proclaiming it would "eliminate waste" and "reduce cost."[9] Where have we heard that recently? The National Health System in Britain, after fifty years, is seeing hospitalized patients die from neglect, more than a million people waiting for surgery, and a general decline in longevity. By their own research, the British published data showing that men in America have a 66 percent average five-year survival from cancer, while British men have only a 45 percent five-year survival—a number that rivals the old Soviet system and is about what men experience with no cancer treatment at all.[10]

Private industry will not produce the products needed for state-of-the-art medicine. We will have more shortages of antibiotics and anesthetic agents and catheters. Doctors will get used to a lesser standard of care, will become blue-collar shift workers, and will no longer concern themselves with caring for their community. They will be too busy trying to save themselves and those close to them. Like the many dispirited Soviet and British physicians, they will simply accept that they are powerless to change the system. Given our present trajectory, this is what awaits us.

5

WHAT THE MELTDOWN WILL LOOK LIKE

Although we can never be certain about the future, events happening now give us some idea of what medicine will be reduced to in the future. In the last chapter I outlined how the accountable care organizations (ACOs) are pushing us toward this future. But even without them, trends are very evident. Today, all over America, small and midsize hospitals as well as hospitals in inner city, poor areas are closing. Recently, Los Angeles Metropolitan Hospital—a 212-bed facility with an emergency room that served the neediest patients—closed. This came in the wake of a federal fraud case citing "unnecessary care" being given to the poor. Although fraud is always a possibility in third-party payment schemes, the truth is that "unnecessary care" is a term used by bureaucrats to avoid paying providers. And quite frankly, as the money has dried up for Medicare and Medicaid, this failure of payment for *actual services rendered* is happening more and more often.

And the result is predictable: economic failure of hospitals and physician practices that have become dependent on government payment for large segments of their population. The hospitals and offices that will close are those with the least private insurance—as in this case of Los Angeles Metropolitan. These closures result in larger and larger areas where no doctors or hospitals exist. As reported in the *Los Angeles Times*, these closures affect small and midsize hospitals "that don't have the negotiating clout or resources of larger hospitals or giant health systems."[1] (This demonstrates a principle of economic fascism known as "cartelization"—businesses joining together into massive cartels to be able to afford the legal and financial advisors needed to navigate the maze of government bureaucracy. Small fry businesses are toast.)

As hospitals close, doctors will move to areas where hospitals are available. In fact, physicians are already preferentially locating to areas where there is a high ratio of private to government insurance.

Malpractice insurance costs also aggravate this flight to more "genteel" areas. The naked truth is doctors are more likely to be sued by the neediest segments of society, as well as those hospitalized for high-level trauma.

At one point (I don't know if this is true today, but it was true when I was an orthopaedic resident visiting Ranchos Los Amigos in the late 1980s) the senior spinal surgeon at Ranchos Los Amigos spinal cord injury center was the most-sued doctor in America and could not buy malpractice insurance at any cost. Was he incompetent? NO. He was arguably one of the handful of the most highly trained, highly experienced surgeons in his field. But his population consisted of indigent trauma and gunshot victims who had been rendered quadriplegic or paraplegic by their injuries but who were angry about their injuries and saw the surgeon as a potential source of money. So, in addition to making less income and having less hospital support, if you practice in an impoverished community, you are more likely to lose your assets to a large malpractice settlement or to exorbitant insurance fees.

The effect of all this is to create huge, expanding black holes where no medical care exists. Already in some areas of Arizona, for the reasons just cited, pregnant women must travel two hundred miles or more to see an obstetrician and to deliver their babies. Needless to say, roadside and in-ambulance births are reported more frequently. And for those in high-risk pregnancy categories, this means increased risk of complications around the time of the birth. A better option for those who can afford it is moving in with relatives or into a hotel near a tertiary care center as their due dates approach.

As hospitals close, the remaining centers and clinics will have insufficient money to expand their services. But at the same time they will be overwhelmed with patients who are coming in from a larger radius and who are taking advantage of the government's funding of "free" preventive care.

So even if you make it to such a center, your wait times may be significant. The hospital in Arizona where I used to work is a 250-bed facility with the latest state-of-the-art cardiac care. It is a referral center for about four hundred thousand people. Although you will get great care there, if you go by foot or car to the emergency room with chest pain, you may wait over six hours for an evaluation because the system is overloaded. In the university hospital in Montreal, gurneys are lined up in the hallways from one end of the building to another, filled with patients waiting for days to be seen in the ER.[2] Ironically, my little twenty-five-bed hospital in the wilds of Iowa has no cardiac program, but if you walk in there with chest pain, you will be evaluated with an EKG that will be reviewed by a physician in fewer than fifteen minutes. You may need to be transferred for definitive care, but you will have immediate and potentially lifesaving support, and the total transport time still is less than the wait time in some big-city ERs. Yet these little hospitals—which serve a vital role in our system today—are the ones falling victim to the government squeeze.

As the money further dries up, more and more facilities will close, and you will have to travel farther and farther for care. This means you will need to anticipate your medical needs further in advance, postpone nonessential care, and decide to treat smaller things at home on your own. (The last half of this book is written to facilitate this self-care.)

A second aspect of the economic squeeze on doctors and hospitals is threefold: it includes the lack of supplies needed to provide care, an inability to provide the latest technology, and the tendency to scrimp on your care to save the facility money.

Recently, the father of the one of my hospital staff experienced recurrent cardiac arrhythmia—irregular heartbeat. He was told by his cardiologist to have an implantable pacemaker/defibrillator, and this recommendation was subsequently confirmed by two other heart specialists. Furthermore, he was advised, in writing, that without this he had a very significant risk of death within two years. In spite of this, an unelected Medicare bureaucrat determined that he did not meet "the minimum criteria" for the implant, because his "cardiac output" was too high. Now, cardiac output is a measure of how well the heart pumps blood. This is significant in other heart disease but has absolutely nothing to do with people who have intermittent arrhythmia. Nevertheless, some nonphysician Health and Human Services pogue[3] consulted the guidelines and refused to authorize the care. But—and this is the kicker—since Medicare had a fee scale for the procedure, my friend's father—a Medicare recipient—*could not buy the procedure privately*. Once you are a Medicare recipient, if Medicare offers the procedure (even if they do not offer it to you), you cannot privately contract for it—at any price—unless you go overseas. I have had similar denials by Tricare, Medicaid, and other government payers. They are not denying care because they—the bureaucrats—really know better than your doctor. Of course they do not. They are denying care because they are trying to save money, and they do it by denying care to some people so they can offer other care to another group.

On the walls of my former hospital was posted the "mission statement," which read, in part, that the hospital's mission was "rational use of resources." In my role as rebel *with* a cause, I pointed out that my Hippocratic oath committed me to do the best for my individual patients, not withhold the hospital's resources at the expense of my patient. "Rational use of resources" makes sense if you are a lightbulb manufacturer. Let's say 100-watt lightbulbs are selling well but 40-watt bulbs are not. It makes sense to "rationally reallocate resources" by shutting down the 40-watt production line in favor of the 100-watt line. But how does this apply to health care? When government or any third party controls the purse, it means they decide to deny care to some to give it to others. Usually this is done on the basis of the utilitarian principle of the greatest good to the greatest number. This dictates, and is practiced in every socialized system of medical care, that the very young and the old are sacrificed as being unproductive in favor of working taxpayers.

Denials of care are couched in terms such as "not medically necessary," "deemed futile," "experimental," or "does not meet standard of care"—none of which may be true. The point is simply to save money, and hospitals can do this only by rationing care. That's all fine and good if you are not the one being rationed! And this is supported by a propaganda program that makes people feel guilty about spending too much on themselves or their aged loved ones.

Recently I was consulted to see an elderly woman with a broken hip. This was a very simple fracture that could be stabilized without even opening the skin except to make three puncture wounds and slip in three threaded titanium screws. I have done hundreds of these, and the actual surgery takes about ten minutes after anesthesia and positioning. Postoperatively, we get people up walking within a day and out of the hospital within three days. Without the surgery, the patient would not be able to walk until (and if) the fracture heals— weeks to months. And of course, for a ninety-year-old, this is often a death sentence, since weakness and the chance of pneumonia go way up in the elderly who quit walking. Nevertheless, the patient's daughter—a nurse—decided that surgery was too aggressive and too much "end of life care" and opted for nursing home placement. And her mother agreed—not wanting to be a burden. Before this the alert patient had been active and living alone on her own. What a tragedy. But this will be the "standard of care" in the future.

Overregulation has resulted in lack of supplies and the latest medications. Cancer drugs are constantly updating as new science improves our treatment options. But Medicare (along with the FDA and other players who caused the inflated prices to begin with) is now trying to save money by denying the use of some of these latest drugs. In many cases they "allow" the use but pay so little for the drugs that the providers cannot afford to dispense them. And patients are prohibited from paying the cash difference to obtain the drug. Some oncologists were actually paying out of pocket to supply these drugs to their patients when it really made a difference.[4] But this could not be sustained for long, and most of these drugs are no longer in general use.

To make matters worse, FDA and OSHA have closed many drug factories by demanding that they bring their old factories "up to today's standards"—something factories producing the cheaper drugs cannot afford to do. The result is lack of basic drugs, such as Armour Thyroid and tetanus vaccine. At a major trauma facility, I was unable to get tetanus toxoid for patients for about two months due to a national shortage. (It is important to keep your tetanus vaccine up to date *before* you get injured because you may not have the vaccine available exactly when you need it. Routinely, ten years is the time that tetanus vaccine is deemed effective. You should consult your physician now and make sure you are up to date on tetanus. Also, discuss with your pharmacist which drugs you take that are at risk of shortage now or in the future. In other words, make sure your medications are not on the "endangered" list. If they are, time to stock up as noted in chapter 15.)

A third aspect of the collapse will be loss of medical records. Already with the government-mandated EMR (electronic medical records), the quality and availability of your medical information has diminished. I know, I know . . . the pointy-headed guys in Washington told you that computerization would solve everything—that no duplication of tests would occur because your doctor would have your whole medical history at the touch of a button. Let me assure you: that assertion is anything but the truth. In fact, on computerized charts it is now much harder to read and understand your history, and working in a clinic today is like practicing medicine with Alzheimer's—with no memory of past events and starting afresh every visit. One of my physician friends with a high-volume ENT practice said to me, "I just hope the patient will say something to remind me who they are and why they are here."

Some of the problems of EMR are simply ones of newness and implementation. But sadly, some problems are intrinsic to computerization. And this fact is lost on one-size-fits-all government guys.

Because there is no "industry standard" EMR, the record generated at hospital A cannot be often accessed by hospital B directly. You may be able to look at it on a CD brought physically (i.e., via "sneaker net") from one hospital to another, but it is unlikely that it will integrate into your current record. (In the old days, paper was universally understood and accessible.)

And then there is the problem of organization. Some EMRs are simply organized chronologically without thought to the type of information being stored. So a patient's EKG is put on top of the orthopaedic visit, which is on top of the list of primary care visits, which are on top of laboratory data. It takes so long to find the *relevant* medical history that doctors do not have time to both find your history and see you in the clinic in the time allotted. Imagine trying to find a file in your computer that has no specific name and is just stored by type and date. Could you do it easily? No. And so to compensate, in my clinic, your entire medical history (which I actually have at my fingertips) is condensed into a one-line handwritten sentence that my office manager places at the top of a clipboard sheet.

A major problem with EMR is its lack of detail. People and their medical problems are analog—displaying infinite variety and complexity. But EMR is digital and finite. A digital record gives you only certain stylized options in recording a patient's history. And although you have the option of dictating segments of the chart, this is often too cumbersome to be practical. So as time goes on, like water flowing to the lowest levels, a physician settles for less and less specific patient history in favor of a generalized, "cookie-cutter" description of the problem. So, for example, instead of a postoperative clinic visit that records the procedure as a "partial medial menisectomy with removal of 25 percent surface area of the meniscus and removal of a small firm plica," the visit is for "post-op knee arthroscopy." As a spinal surgeon, sometimes I need a neurologist to render an opinion on whether the patient's problem stems from the spinal compression (stenosis) or from a more metabolic sickness of the nerves (polyneuropathy). In the old days of paper, I used to get dictated reports back from my neurologic consultant that outlined his reasoning and gave me a feel for the more probable answer. Now I get a digital summary that simply states "stenosis" and "polyneuropathy," with CPT codes attached. So the patient is poorer—having just paid for a fairly useless consult—and I am no wiser, still unable to determine if surgery is likely to help him. Needless to say, I rarely ask for such consults anymore.

And then there is the issue of accuracy. The old saying "garbage in, garbage out" is as true with medical records as with any other computer function. It is very time-consuming to input the data required to set up a new patient chart, so clinic secretaries use cut and paste, taking snips from all the other records to make the new record. Of course, in the interim since that old data was generated, the patient may have been hospitalized and had major changes to his history and medications. The easier it is to hit a key and replicate old information, the easier it is to pass on falsehoods.

Is it any coincidence that Epic, the largest EMR system, was designed by one of Obama's largest financial backers? Epic may be better than some, but it still decreases quality of care and makes doctors inefficient. There are all sorts of PR programs and rah-rah teams to convince us how great this is—signs around our facility say "We're EPIC strong!" In contrast, PACS, the digital Radiology system designed by and for doctors years ago was an immediate hit because it solved problems we wanted solved, was high quality, and made us *more* efficient. We didn't need cheerleaders to sell it to us.

The upshot of all this is that you will not be able to trust your health to this Orwellian medical record system. (See appendix D for detailed instructions on creating your own personal medical record that is optimized for the people who will be caring for you regularly or in an emergency.)

So what will the meltdown look like? There will be large wastelands where no organized medical care exists. You will be discouraged at all levels from high-level care, as most doctors will be working, not for you, but for the government and will be only too happy to do the bureaucrats' bidding by denying you care—either overtly or covertly (by not making you aware of the latest medical options available). Supplies and medicines will be in shorter and shorter supply. You will not have the luxury of your doctor or hospital keeping accurate, accessible medical records for you. In short, you will be more and more on your own for yourself and your family. A good understanding of the endgame is found in Yuri Maltsev's article, "What Soviet Medicine Teaches Us" (see appendix A).

When I debate socialists on health care, they object to being compared to the Soviet Union, but Soviet-style medicine is the endgame. It represents all the philosophy of today's government health care proponents rolled into one great, disastrous experiment. If we cannot learn from that, what lesson can we learn?

6

THE ROLE OF INSURANCE

As the government consumes what is left of private practice medicine, the role of insurance becomes less clear. Recently, I gave a speech to medical students. Afterwards I was approached by one of the students who said, "I have never heard of catastrophic insurance." I'm sure the student paid for *car insurance*, but because there is no crisis in car insurance, she didn't give a thought as to how car insurance actually works. It is a sad fact that—thanks to the perversion of the free marketplace by government and corrupt insurance companies—we have raised a generation of young people who do not understand how *real insurance* works. They believe they have health insurance. In reality, what they purchase today in medicine is not insurance but "prepaid health care."

Real insurance functions like this: For any given problem, a special mathematical genius called an actuary figures out the probability of some problem occurring to an individual subscriber. The actuary uses a person's demographics, and can predict the probability of accident and project the cost of that accident or disease. For example, an actuary can tell me my probability of totaling my car. He has a vast array of statistics, can look up the data about middle-aged women driving sports cars, and knows that generally we are harmless compared to young men armed with the same fast car. So my premiums are lower than my son would pay for the same coverage. Car insurance and house insurance are referred to as actuarial-based insurance. Neither government nor special-interest groups have skewed the market, so the cost is generally low, and coverage is typically understandable and predictable.

Furthermore, regarding your car insurance, you, not your employer, own it. It is, therefore, infinitely portable. You can choose how much or how little to self-insure, and what you want covered. You can buy it across state lines in a big national market. In sum, for all of these reasons, those types of insurance are not in crisis.

Health insurance, before Medicare and the more recent government meddling, was functional and cheaper in the same way. When it worked it was known as "major medical" insurance—a form of catastrophic, actuarial-based insurance. Most outpatient care was paid out of pocket. Insurance kicked in *only* for big-ticket items. When you saw a physician for things such as well child care, vaccinations, a runny nose, a routine checkup, and so forth, you paid cash because this fell outside actuarial probability. But when you got hospitalized and had surgery to remove your gallbladder, insurance kicked in.

Insurance companies, years ago, found they could woo customers by offering to pay for "trinkets" such as glasses, wellness, and outpatient testing. Patients, acting in their own self-interest, got more for their insurance dollar by availing themselves of these things, so they used their insurance to the greatest extent possible. Insurance companies then had to raise fees to cover costs, and it created a downward spiral of overutilization and failed attempts at cost containment. When it morphed to this prepaid health care, medical insurance became the only insurance we *wanted to use*. Think about your other insurance. Really, you hope you never need to use your home or auto insurance. When you need those insurances to kick in, it means something bad has happened. And that notion used to be true for health insurance—before big insurance companies wanted to be all things to all people and before special-interest groups used the power of government to mandate insurance coverage of things such as mammograms.

Predictably, this approach to medical insurance has fueled escalating medical prices. It goes like this: An MRI costs $400 for cash. But then a screening MRI for some illness is mandated for coverage by the government. Now the MRI center must bill an insurance company and wait thirty days or more to get paid, so it increases the cost of the screening to $500 to cover its administrative overhead and late payments. The insurance company is having trouble with covering its costs because suddenly there is an increased utilization in MRIs that its actuaries did not factor in when computing insurance premiums. And the company cannot raise premiums on a daily basis to adjust, so it stalls payment and denies claims. This adds more administrative burden to the MRI center, which hires more staff to deal with the paperwork of disputed claims and which writes off more for nonpayment. Now it has to charge $1,000 per study to make an operating profit. Then the insurance premiums are raised. And this spiral continues without end.

Think what would happen to your car insurance if it covered oil changes and every little ding in your paint.

The solution to this problem, both on a national level and on a personal level, is to return to real, actuarial-based insurance. Today this is generally called "high-deductible" insurance. And the higher the deductible ($2,500 to $10,000), generally the better coverage you have when you are sick. It means you pay for most outpatient items, and insurance kicks in for the "big-ticket" illnesses and accidents. Think about your home insurance. When a shingle blows off, you don't call your insurance agent. You reach into your pocket and pay for a new shingle and probably put it on yourself. (You don't reach into your neighbor's pocket, either, by the way.) When your roof blows off, *then* you call your insurance for help.

The saddest side effect of prepaid health care is the confusion and lack of transparency. It is nearly impossible to know what you are actually paying for and what you will really be covered for if you fall ill. This confusion is a direct result of insurance companies' vain attempts at cost containment by writing a million little rules to curb overutilization. In some cases this is abject fraud as they game play to avoid payment to hospitals and providers. (At one point, according to an insurance whistle-blower, a major insurance company shredded every third claim in its mailroom to stall payment.) And it is a result of uncertainty. In my office I could determine my monthly overhead down to the penny. But no matter how many contracts I signed, how many agreements I made, or how many people I talked to, I could never know how much I would be paid for a procedure or office visit. I never knew when I was getting paid from month to month. I never knew if the government or Blue Cross would write to me years hence and ask for the money back saying they had determined they had overpaid me or that the care I rendered was "unnecessary."

Imagine if that were how you bought tomatoes. You told the grocer, "I'm taking the tomatoes but not paying you. Charge my insurance company, and they may or may not pay you. And if they decide to pay you, it may take you a year to get paid." Can you imagine what that would do to the price of tomatoes? Do you understand why there is a lack of "transparency in pricing"? The cost of tomatoes is relatively low and stable, and you know how much tomatoes cost because you pay cash at the time of service. When you are paying for medical care through a third party, the third party may agree to one price but pay another. Doctors routinely sign contracts with insurance companies that are then violated as insurance companies and Medicare delay payment, underpay, or pay and then years later ask for all or part of the money back. How could a grocer, or any business, function within such a scenario? It can't and we can't—for long.

Buying high-deductible insurance and paying cash for the little stuff is generally much better. When you are hospitalized or need a study, such as a blood test or CT scan, then your deductible insurance kicks in. Period. Little guesswork. One of the secrets is to negotiate all cash prices. Prices are set to reflect the insanity of the prepaid health care system. But if you are paying cash for a procedure or a pill or a doctor's visit, you are relieving the provider of mountains of paperwork and an indeterminate wait for their money. Doctors and hospitals cannot by law charge less than Medicare rates, but Medicare rates often are acceptable if the provider can get the cash at the time of service and can circumvent all the office time to bill a third party.

In recent years, many people believed they could not afford health care when they actually could—at least before Obamacare kicked in. *Individual plans* were usually much cheaper than group, employer-based plans. A problem with group plans is they must cover everything for everybody. Therefore the sixty-year-old woman is paying for prenatal care and for pregnancy care, which she does not need. Before Obamacare, a twenty-five-year-old man with no medical problems could buy health insurance for less than $150 a month. Of course, it was much cheaper before the advent of Obamacare, which has already increased nearly everyone's policy and made the "market" completely unpredictable.

I have been impacted in many ways by PPACA (or, to give credit where credit is due, "Obamacare"). But the most stunning attack on my person came recently in the form of insurance rate hikes. My older son is twenty-four, a medical student, and in perfect health. He has never smoked, is thin, has totally normal labs, is on no meds, and comes from a long line of hearty, healthy stock. It seemed appropriate to pay $47 a month for health insurance, which I have done for over a year now. Then, last month, I received notice from Coventry Insurance that, due to the new health care law, we had to make a choice from three options: (1) we could keep his insurance policy and pay four times as much—$167/month, (2) we could explore a different "ACA compatible" policy, or (3) we could try our luck at the Iowa "marketplace"—i.e., the Obamacare state exchange.

Each option had its own phone number.

Now, honestly, I'd rather sell my kid into indentured labor than put him on Obamacare, so I called the number for the new policy.

I did the appropriate button pushing but ended up at the state exchange. And I confess: after a short conversation with a probable navigator, I hung up, saying there was no way I wanted Obamacare. I also confess that I may have been a bit abrupt in my approach, thinking I would never talk to him again. So I dialed the number for option 1—updating the original policy.

To my horror I again landed in the proverbial lap of the same phone navigator—is there only one of these guys for the whole state? So now, I asked more questions, and discovered the dirty little secret about those three options: there are *not* three insurance options. There is really only one option and only one possible policy. The *only* "option" is whether the great state of Iowa or I will be paying the premium!

So let's be clear. A policy once costing $47 a month—a price many young people or their parents could afford—is now made vastly more expensive ($167 per month), but the price tag is being picked up for the "poor" at the same inflated price by the State of Iowa.

Am I the only one who sees a basic flaw in this scenario? I, one of the few remaining taxpayers, will be paying four times as much for my own insurance and paying taxes for state-subsidized insurance. And this "insurance" for the poor is also four times the actual market value. So, unless I choose to be an underworking deadbeat and go on the government dole myself, I lose financially on every front.

And remember that ACA is an acronym standing for—my fingers are cramping just typing this—the *Affordable* Care Act.

Don't think these increased premiums are increasing any payment to the hospitals and doctors who care for you. We are all taking big cuts. Small hospitals all over the country are teetering on the brink of financial ruin.

Remember when Obama said you could "keep your doctor"? What he really meant was, you may have to actually keep your doctor—like, in your basement. And you may need to bring in a few unemployed hospital administrators and nurses as well.

The reason for this outrageous price hike is what insurance insiders refer to as the 1:3 rule, a regulation in PPACA created by a government economic brainchild that specifies that the ratio of cost for an insurance policy written to the lowest rated age group (20s) and the highest rated age group (60–64) can be no more than 300 percent.

I'm sure those lovable pranksters in DC wrote and thought in reverse, thinking they could limit the cost to the elderly by limiting the rates of the elderly to three times the rates of the young. But of course, insurance companies—companies filled with actual thinkers—realized immediately that they could meet the letter of the law simply by forcing young people to pay through the nose for insurance that should be quite a bit cheaper (to wit, 400 percent cheaper!). No wonder insurance companies lobbied hard for Obamacare. Wouldn't you love the government to step in and force people to pay 400 percent of the real cost of some product you create . . . and to make ownership of the product mandatory?!

Unless common sense, the free market, and the rule of law are reintroduced into America—and what is the chance?—we shall probably be forced to divide the twenty-first-century into BO (before Obamacare) and AO (after Obamacare). Using that system, one of the real problems of the BO era was the fifty-five-year-old individual who lost his insurance when he lost his job. He had some established (preexisting) disease and could not get or could not afford a new insurance policy. This truly was a problem created by employer-based health insurance. Had that person lived at an earlier time BO—say, 1952—and bought private insurance as a twenty-year-old, he would have paid premiums for thirty-five years and during that thirty-five years would have used very little of the insurance money on health care. The insurance company would have made money on that patient during those early years and would have invested the funds. Then the insurance company would have been able to afford the actuarially predicted payouts as the patient got older. The patient would not have lost his insurance by losing his job because he owned and had total control over the conditions of his policy. Of course, this required a modicum of personal responsibility, as does any enterprise or activity in a free society. Freedom entails personal responsibility, and the consequence of failure (in the absence of personal responsibility and failing to be responsible) is a problem for the individual. In a free society you cannot act irresponsibly and force your neighbors to pick up the tab.

In our society today, people with preexisting conditions who have lost their employer-based health care are falling into a huge crack, and they have limited options. If they are indigent, they qualify in most states for a form of Medicaid with new rules dictated by the ACA legislation. This can be good for some and worse for others. In Tennessee, for example, under the BO Medicaid rules, a single mother with a child could qualify for Medicaid with an income 400 percent of the poverty level, but a man could not qualify unless he was below the poverty level. So when, in year one AO, the requirement was changed so men could now qualify at 100 percent of the poverty level, men did better; but women who now also qualify at 100 percent of the poverty level were worse off. And let's face it, where are most of the children of single parents domiciled? With the mother. The deep thinkers in DC strike again.

If you are not indigent, or are technically indigent but of the mind-set not to be dependent on government care (good for you), you can be very clever and start your own company group insurance. So, for example, you lose your job but take up selling fire extinguishers or working several part-time jobs or selling Amway. You become your own corporation, hire another family member who also needs insurance, and then buy "group" insurance—for the two of you—and this is guaranteed issue in all states, regardless of your preexisting conditions. Unfortunately you are now hit in the face with the new rates, which can be considerably more than you would have paid for the same or better insurance BO.

On a practical level today, I would urge you to seek out a single-family or single-person insurance policy that you can afford, with a high deductible. If you combine this policy with an HSA (health savings account) or you buy it through your own corporation, you have the best of all worlds. The health savings account allows you to put money tax-free into an account to cover the deductible. The corporation allows you to pay for the insurance with "pretax dollars," so it effectively lowers the cost of the insurance.

If you have employer-based health insurance, to avoid spiraling costs and to avoid the problem of portability, it might be best to own your own policy—but currently you cannot convert directly. Perhaps, someday it will be possible to convert your employer policy to a self-directed, personally owned policy within the same insurance company if you are older. But this is not available today even if, within the same company such as Blue Cross, the employer-based insurance and the single individual insurance are completely separate—it is as if they were two separate companies. So if you lose your job, the fact that you were insured for years with a medical insurance company through your employer does not help you get private insurance through that same insurance firm.

If you are young and healthy, you definitely should consider private, single-party insurance. Some employers will simply put the money back into your paycheck. As an employer I found out I was paying $800 for an employee's insurance that she could buy for less than $400 for herself. You might make money on the deal by switching.

People in my age bracket got hurt the least by the cost of private insurance under Obamacare. I just purchased health insurance de novo. (I started over.) I am a sixty-one-year-old, healthy, nonsmoking female with a little need for thyroid support and intermittent inhalers for bronchospasm. I was able to purchase health insurance with a $5,000 deductible for under $367 a month (albeit my quote BO was under $200 a month). There is no free lunch. But this does not strike me as exorbitant considering what I am getting for it.

If in the future the government outlaws all private care and makes government the "single payer," then insurance will become meaningless. But in any country that allows a two-tiered system as England has had, real catastrophic, high-deductible, understandable, actuarial-based insurance is still the best way to go.

PART II
GETTING PREPARED

7

ADDICTION

O bviously, the most important thing you can do to survive a medical care meltdown is to be so healthy and safety conscious that you will not need a doctor's intervention. It is beyond the scope of this book to educate the reader about all aspects of wellness, but in appendix A you will find a reference list for further reading that is well worth the time and effort to work through if you want to maximize your health.

Regardless of your current health, there are several things that are basic to wellness. I will outline these, then provide a clear strategy for attaining optimal health based on the latest science.

I don't need to outline the risk of disease from smoking, chewing tobacco, or doing harmful drugs—do I? And if you are a smoker, you are already finding the cost of your habit getting higher and higher. But imagine for a moment a time in the future when suddenly your supply chain of your addictive substance is cut off. Imagine if you woke up today and could not get a cigarette anywhere at any price because of an economic collapse. How would you feel? Now, imagine going through withdrawal from cigarettes or drugs (even legal, prescription ones) at a time when there is no food in the stores. When you should be worried about your children getting enough to eat, instead you are focused on your own physical withdrawal from cigarettes or alcohol or some other addictive substance. America is approaching a 300 percent debt-to-GDP (gross domestic product) ratio. No country has lasted for more than a few years at that level without experiencing a severe economic "readjustment" (less politely, a "collapse"). At such a time in the future, you will need all your wits focused on day-to-day survival. You cannot afford to be "jonesing," as you are suddenly forced into abstinence from your habit. It is far better to stop now in a controlled environment than to suddenly be forced to withdraw from the habit due to collapse of the economy.

Regarding cigarettes, I suspect, too, that American socialized health care will significantly discriminate against tobacco users, even denying some treatment options to smokers as being "futile." And of course, tobacco vastly increases your risk of cancer, heart disease, bone fragility, and other aspects of premature aging. You cannot afford to increase your dependence on a medical system that will no longer be able to respond to your needs.

Ditto for anyone addicted to alcohol. Time to clean up this act. Not every alcoholic experiences the withdrawal symptoms known as DTs or delirium tremens—a very serious disruption of normal body function with skyrocketing blood pressure, increased heart rate, sweating, total body itching, and hallucinations. In the old days, before modern medicine, DTs were 50 percent fatal. The fatalities often were from hallucinations that caused the alcoholic to jump from a hospital window. Again, you don't want to have this happen to you suddenly because the supply of alcohol is unexpectedly disrupted. (You can't get your "still" working in the three days it takes to experience DTs or other withdrawal symptoms.) You don't have to give up the occasional martini or the dinner glass of wine. But you must give up the excess.

Everything I just wrote about alcohol also applies to people who regularly take antianxiety drugs, such as Xanax or Valium. Sudden withdrawal of these drugs—in the family known as *benzodiaz-epines*—may cause you to experience delirium tremens just as you would during withdrawal from alcohol. You cannot suddenly stop such medications. While time permits, discuss with your doctor how to get off all substances that—if suddenly stopped—will produce physical, not just emotional, withdrawal. If, for example, you take Xanax for anxiety, your doctor can *slowly* wean you off and replace it with something that won't give you DTs if suddenly stopped. Yes, you may have to live with depression if medication is not available in a meltdown, but you won't be dying from withdrawal. If, for medical reasons, you cannot stop the drugs, then you must ensure an adequate supply. I will discuss that in the chapter on stockpiling medications, but keep in mind that storing thyroid medications is easier to do than building up a stockpile of highly controlled substances that are closely monitored because they are subject to being diverted from real patients and sold in the street drug trade.

Coffee has many healthful effects, and caffeine in small doses has benefits to daily life and sports performance. But if you are a caffeine junkie who cannot go without that morning jolt and continue to jolt yourself through the day with sixteen cups of java—you might be laid low should your supply dry up. Slowly wean yourself down to one to two cups of coffee or caffeinated "power drinks" a day. A sudden withdrawal of caffeine will give you days to months of headaches and can precipitate severe constipation.

In sum, if you are addicted to anything—psychologically or physically, consider what would happen in an economic collapse when for three to six months you had no chance to obtain your substance of choice. I don't really care what the addiction is—it could be Krispy Kreme donuts—although some substances are clearly more dangerous to stop precipitously than others. It is much better to wean yourself off these substances slowly before the meltdown. In a mass economic shutdown, keep in mind you will not be the only one involved, and medical facilities will quickly be overrun with people out of their medications and their addictive substances. If alcohol is your problem, if you smoke or chew, or you use any other addictive substance—deal with it now. Consult your physician and/or support groups, such as Alcoholics Anonymous or the local smoking cessation organization.

I am always amused by people who smoke and take vitamins. I once gave a talk on health to a group of government workers. To make my point I showed a cartoon of a safe falling from a second-story window. In the cartoon, a man is walking down the street and is looking down at a wad of chewing gum, being very careful not to get it on his shoe, while above him a safe is hurtling down on his head. The gum was labeled "supplements," and the safe was labeled "smoking." I think you get the point. Before worrying about diet, exercise, or supplements, you must eliminate the problems that are *really bad*. Do it now.

8

DIET: WHAT SCIENCE REALLY TELLS US

Thereis nothing more important to your health than a good, "clean" diet. A good diet—and I am going to define this clearly—will give you the best chance of surviving the medical meltdown. I don't want you to *need* a doctor who isn't there. In this chapter, after explaining all the reasons *not* to eat in certain ways, I will give you a summary of a "clean," optimized diet. But my advice is to read it all. This is probably the most important prevention chapter in this book. The more you understand the *reasons* behind dietary recommendations, the more you will be psychologically invested in eating correctly.

You literally are what you eat. Eat crap, become crap. Unfortunately, what we think of as food in many cases is so artificial it bears no resemblance to *real* food. Would your great-grandmother have recognized boxed macaroni and cheese as something to eat? Leave a Twinkie open in your car for six months and it won't look much different from the day you opened the package. Why? Because even bacteria don't recognize it as food! In my home state of Iowa, we joke about the traditional meat-and-potatoes diet. But in the days when my ancestors homesteaded on the prairie, they ate nothing from boxes. They ate all sorts of meat, with its fat, vegetables from the garden, some corn, real milk from cows, butter, lard, and the few nuts and berries that grew wild here. And in my great-grandparents' and grandparents' generations, people who were not felled by childhood diseases routinely lived into their nineties. After World War II, enter agribusiness, donut shops, and hot dogs, and we think seventy-five years old is beating the odds.

WHAT HAPPENS BETWEEN MOUTH AND RECTUM

When you eat any substance (I am avoiding calling everything we put in our mouths food), that material is broken down and absorbed by your intestines (gut). These particles are sorted by the very sophisticated cells in your gut to determine if they should be taken in or pooped out (excreted as feces). Once the particles are selected for absorption, they flow through the bloodstream and are deposited in various parts of the body, including the liver, the brain, and your muscles. Let me stop there. I want you to think about what I just said. Everything you eat ends up in your blood and your brain. Before reaching for that terrible, totally artificial, red dye no. 23–infused, sugarcoated, no-nutrition candy—consider that it is going to flow through your bloodstream and land in your brain! *We worry about polluting our water supply. Time to worry about polluting our blood supply.*

Back to the metabolic process: These food (and nonfood) particles are absorbed into the various cells and, through metabolism, are processed into the building blocks that become you. And you are constantly being updated and replaced. Every two years you are nearly a totally different person, as the old cells have been replaced by new cells. So if you are fat, diabetic, and out of shape, just remember the words of screenwriter and film director Cameron Crowe: "Every passing minute is another chance to turn it all around."[1]

Now, the world of food and obesity is much more complex than "calorie in, calorie out." Some foods produce fat, some raise your insulin and blood sugar, and some do not—even if they are high calorie. When I eat sugar or wheat, I am eating pure carbo-hydrates at four calories a gram. When I eat a lean venison steak, I am getting almost pure protein and also four calories a gram, but there is a big difference. The sugar and wheat cause my insulin to shoot up. Insulin is a hormone that signals my cells to deposit the carbohydrate calories as fat. With prolonged ingestion of such carbohydrates, my cells will become insulin resistant, meaning the receptors on my cells reject insulin unless it is forced onto the cell in high concentration. As I become progressively "insulin resistant," my body produces more and more insulin to compensate, and it is still never enough to keep blood sugar normal, so I become diabetic. Protein does not raise insulin, so rather than being stored as fat, it is metabolized to energy and helps me build muscle.

So what happens when I eat fat? Well, as you will read later—a lot of good things. But for right now, just understand that fat has nine calories per gram, but it does not raise insulin and, by itself, does not get deposited as fat. The Inuit were a lean, mean, muscular people when they ate a diet consisting of 90 percent blubber (whale fat). Then the European explorers brought with them processed grains and—kablooey! The Inuit, who had survived thousands of years of bone-numbing cold and polar bears and whale hunting, were laid low by obesity and the diseases of modern civilization. Ancient man had a chronically low level of insulin because he was not surrounded by, and not eating, carbohydrate-laden foods. And as the science of nutrition progresses, we recognize that high insulin levels are at the heart of our metabolic derangements. Fat has gotten a terrible rap, but in fact, when you eat fat, the absorption of simultaneously ingested carbohydrates is slowed, thereby limiting the bad insulin spikes. This explains the counterintuitive fact that skim milk is much worse for spiking insulin than full-cream milk; ditto low-fat yogurt versus full-fat, Greek yogurt; low-fat ice cream versus the real deal. Another big advantage of fat—it fills you up. It makes you want to stop eating. And—witness French cooking—it is damn tasty! Put this together and it goes a long way to explaining why, since Americans have been told to eat low fat, we have become fatter and sicker.

The point is, all calories are not the same. It is not just simple "input to output." To optimize our health, we need to eat correctly to make the ancient metabolic process we inherited over the generations work properly. Think of your body as a Porsche that has been fine-tuned to perform perfectly on high-octane, water-free fuel. When the Porsche is fed good gas, it purrs along with power and keeps running with minimal preventive maintenance. In life, we see these "Porsche people" as strong, slender, active, and clear thinking. Think of the old Sioux or Apache warriors—muscled, lean, and standing fiercely and cleverly against the injustice they faced. Think of the natural body builders, of Jack LaLanne at ninety-two, doing fingertip pushups. That's based on clean dietary habits.

What happens if you routinely "feed" the Porsche low-octane, poor-quality gas? It stutters and loses power, and you'll be in for expensive car repair sooner than expected. Giving the Porsche bad gas is the equivalent of the Native American of today eating flour tortillas and cheesy puffs and white rice. The once-healthy Southwest Indians now have the highest rate of diabetes in the world and are generally dead by age fifty-five. Bad gas in a sports car can cause sludge to build up in the engine. When people eat a terrible, artificial, cheap-carbohydrate, Western diet, before their insulin shoots up they have spikes of relatively high blood glucose. During those times, they deposit sugar molecules onto their cells—in their brains, in their blood cells, and in their muscles. This process, called *glycation*, alters their tissues so that they cannot function optimally and ultimately fail early. Think of your healthy cell as a runner and your glycated cell as a runner dragging a fifty-pound weight behind him as he tries to run. Every glycated cell in the body is made less effective, including the cells that fight infection and the brain cells that think.

The second aging process caused by bad diet is "oxidation"— literally a rusting of the tissues. Oxidation is produced by the metabolic process of converting your food to energy. In the Porsche, think of it as the exhaust from your engine. A little bit of pollutant exhaust is inevitable, and in the body, a little bit of free oxygen radical production is normal; but these potentially damaging radicals are neutralized by "antioxidants" produced in the cells. Eat a good diet and your antioxidant production goes up, your production of oxygen radicals is only moderate, and you have more than enough antioxidant capability to neutralize them. Eat a bad diet and the opposite happens: you produce too many free oxygen radicals for the body to neutralize, so they run free and literally cause the body to rust. Rusting of metal is oxidation; rusting of the body is aging. Outward manifestations of body oxidation (rusting) are age spots, sagging, and diminished luminance of the skin.

A bad, Western-style, high-carb diet also causes whole-body *inflammation*. We hear a lot about inflammation, mostly when discussing the term *anti-inflammatory*. But what is inflammation, really? Inflammation is an immune system process designed to fight infection. Get a splinter and you will see inflammation at work. In medical training we learn the four cardinal signs of inflammation are redness, heat, pain, and swelling. (Well, we learn them in Latin: *rubor, calor, dolor,* and *tumor*—because they rhyme and because it gives us yet another chance to sound erudite and pompous.) Inflammation results from your immune cells waging war against the foreign object or germ. The cells surround the invader and release chemicals that cause swelling, pain, heat, or redness (the four cardinal signs). This reaction is meant to be a local phenomenon of short duration. But a bad diet creates generalized, perpetual, never-ending, whole-body inflammation. The effects of this inflammation range from rheumatoid arthritis to dementia. The so-called diseases of modern civilization—diabetes, heart disease, dementia, and cancer—truly are a result of modern civilization—specifically our modern diet.

WHO DO YOU TRUST?

The first step in eating correctly is to *absolutely forget any government recommendation you have ever heard about what to eat.* And don't buy the nihilist argument that the recommendations change every day. Although your newspaper may be confusing, real science has been consistently zeroing in on an optimal diet for longevity and health. You just don't hear about it in the government-controlled (or at least government-sympathetic and gullible) media. Real nutrition is complicated science, and it takes some education in science to be able to write about it intelligently. Regrettably, real "science writers" who can understand and separate the *probable truth* from the *random idea or fad* are few and far between.

Nor will you get truth from the companies that want to sell you junk food. And when there is a lot of money riding on an idea—even a bad one—it is difficult for the truth to be known. When I was in biochemistry at the University of Rochester in 1976, I remember a lecture on lipid membranes in which I was taught that *ingested cholesterol bore no relationship to blood cholesterol levels.* This turns out to be true. Nevertheless, until very recently the loudest voices, and the ad campaigns, were all against eating cholesterol because—they claimed—it would raise serum cholesterol, and that was bad with a capital *B*. So we have assiduously avoided foods such as eggs, which, it turns out, are just about the most perfect human food. (The cholesterol myth will be debunked later.)

And then there are the special-interest groups, such as PETA, who have their own agendas. The recommendations of such groups are colored by beliefs that put animal welfare above human health. And ironically, they don't even understand animal nutrition correctly. In short, be very suspicious of dietary recommendations that are part of a political agenda or that promote an agribusiness's bottom line.

And keep in mind that the "medical establishment"—the guys who speak with authority in the news—are usually way behind the freethinking leading edge of medicine, the doctors often reviled by the establishment. As a historical point, President Eisenhower was essentially killed by his cardiologists' recommendations to eat vegetable oils rather than natural oils, to avoid cholesterol, and to eat a low-fat, high-carb diet. I know this is the diet that was sold to you as "healthy," the details of which you have probably heard all your life (unless you are lucky enough to know a doctor truly up on the science). But trust me: as we get into the details, you will see that such recommendations have killed countless people over the years and, in general, are to be ignored.

How about nutritionists? With all due respect to the good-guy "nutritionists," in general, today's nutritionists are not getting the latest science. My son, who is in medical school, showed me his online nutrition lecture. It was *so* out of date. In fact, its content in 2013 was out of date when I was in medical school biochemistry in 1976. Sadly, the nutritionists have drunk the government and groupthink Kool-Aid. How do I know I am right and they are wrong? In addition to reading the scientific body of knowledge from multiple sources, I also have an understanding of basic physiology. But mostly, I just need to observe my patients' food to decide who is right. Every day, when I come upon a pile of pancakes, sugary syrup, margarine, and wheat toast on some hospitalized *diabetic* patient's plate—a diet prescribed by the nutrition department—I see the world of nutritionists as the Flat Earth Society. Fortunately, my son, after showing me the abysmal nutrition lecture, said, "I know, Mom. I won't eat that way—just gotta pass the test." Smart lad.

WITH ALL DUE RESPECT—AVOID VEGETARIANISM

Although it is totally politically incorrect to attack the "sacred cow" (excuse the humor) of vegetarianism, I must do it. One of the diets that never seems to go away in spite of the overwhelming evidence against it is *vegetarianism* or the extreme form, *veganism*. While some people eat a vegetarian diet out of religious conviction, many do it under the belief that they are improving their health. Unfortunately, such a diet—no matter how carefully you micromanage your components—simply is inadequate in both micro and macronutrients. Some of the unhealthiest patients I have had in my medical practice believed in eating no meat out of some conviction—either religious, a belief in not killing animals, or their mistaken understanding of the best path to health. It is not my place to question their religious or moral conviction, but I must point out the flawed belief that it is a healthy diet.

For years I cared for a woman in her forties with a multitude of orthopaedic problems. She was pear shaped, looked very pale, had little muscle, and was a strict vegan. When I asked her as politely as I could why she chose to eat this way, she told me that she just could not abide "the thought of hurting animals." Initially, she came to see me for mid back pain and generalized achiness, and I found that she had become kyphotic—curved forward in the upper spine. Her spine X-rays looked like those of a seventy-five-year-old. Her bone density was terribly low, and there was evidence of small wedge compression fractures of the spine bones due to low bone density. We tested her blood, and she proved to be typical of the vegan patients I see in my orthopaedic practice who are almost universally deficient in vitamin D_3 and the B vitamins and generally weak of muscle and bone.

Based on this and the characteristic appearance of her X-rays, I am sure—even without a bone biopsy—that her bone density problem was not just osteoporosis (loss of bone volume) but adult rickets—soft abnormal bone—due to vitamin D_3 deficiency. I placed her on numerous supplements and medicine to improve her bone quality but could never get on top of things. Her energy was low, so exercise was a painful and frustrating experience. She was having frequent diarrhea—probably due to gluten sensitivity—and this added malabsorption to the picture. Her belly fat—another product of her high-carb diet—was distorting her hormonal balance, and she was becoming prediabetic. After she suffered a spontaneous fracture of her foot bone, I had a frank discussion in which I told her she was killing herself with her diet, and although I could keep applying "orthopaedic Band-Aids," it wasn't the way to go.

Unfortunately, her emotional commitment to her diet, formed by her worldview, caused her to choose to continue along her path of rapid functional decline.

As reported in a study in the *Annals of Nutrition and Metabolism*, B_{12} deficiency ranges from 20 percent in semi-vegetarians to 92 percent in vegans.[2] In other words, the stricter the meatlessness, the more deficient you become in this critical vitamin. B_{12} is vital, not only to building the blood, but to nerve and brain health. For example, it was discovered, using sophisticated studies of B_{12} blood levels, that 30 percent of men with dementia are B_{12} deficient. And in another study, people with low vitamin B_{12} levels were at double the risk of developing Alzheimer's disease (in 370 elderly men and women followed over three years).[3] In my practice I sometimes cure cases of polyneuropathy (dysfunction of the nerves) by giving people sublingual (under the tongue) supplementation of B_{12}, even when their labs are reported as "normal." In sum, B_{12} is critical and simply cannot be guaranteed on a vegetarian diet.

Creatine and animal protein in the right ratios likewise are deficient in vegetarians. This leads to weakness and to measurable deficiency in muscle mass.[4] Bodybuilders and weight lifters of all kinds (myself included) take creatine to improve muscle gains. And it is my observation, while snowboarding with friends and working on the farm, that vegetarians simply do not have the stamina or strength of those of us who eat meat.

Additionally, vegetarianism leads to deficiencies in vitamin D_3.[5] Vitamin D is not a vitamin but a hormone that is, in my opinion, the cheapest anti-aging pill we have. Vitamin D_3 deficiency has been associated with childhood rickets—a bone disorder—for more than a hundred years. And it has been known since the 1970s that those living on the equator, where they get an abundance of vitamin D_3 from exposure to the sun, regardless of particular locale, have lower rates of multiple sclerosis, colon cancer, and depression. But more recently, many astute observers have discovered that low vitamin D_3 leads to many other disorders, including adult rickets, cardiac arrhythmias, breast cancer, adult fractures, dementia, heart attacks, and even diabetes.

Most recently, studies have demonstrated that higher levels of vitamin D_3 improve longevity and are beneficial at preventing influenza—even better than vaccination.[6] Studies showing the beneficial effects of high vitamin D_3 levels are quite convincing. They not only show a correlation between low vitamin D_3 blood levels and the medical problem in question, but they also show improvement in the disease or prevention of the condition when levels are raised through supplementation. And I have seen patients feel better in two weeks after starting vitamin D_3 supplementation. At first I was skeptical that this was a placebo effect, but I have seen it too many times to believe this now. I do not know the mechanism of the sudden improvement, but I suspect these people have critically low initial blood levels because of diet, lack of sunlight and use of sunscreens, northern latitude, and so forth.

It has been shown in the laboratory that heart muscle does not contract well unless adequate vitamin D_3 is present. An Italian population study showed that low vitamin D_3 levels were proportional to atherosclerotic plaques (clogging of the arteries).[7] Furthermore, a Japanese study of dialysis patients demonstrated that correcting vitamin D_3 deficiency significantly lowered death rate from heart attacks and heart disease in general.[8] This is only a snapshot of the rapidly expanding body of literature supporting the role of vitamin D_3 in prevention of multiple diseases. But to achieve the positive effects, blood levels of D_3 need to be in the range of 50 to 100 nanograms per deciliter, not the 20 nanograms per deciliter that laboratories report as the lowest range of "normal." Specifically in the case of breast cancer, if one achieves blood levels above 50 nanograms per deciliter, the risk of breast cancer is diminished 83 percent.[9] This is not surprising, because vitamin D_3 works at a very basic level keeping telomeres—the ends of our DNA strands—healthy. Studies of equatorial inhabitants demonstrate that some of the longest-lived people on the planet obtain 30,000 to 40,000 international units of vitamin D (specifically D_3) a day from the sunlight—nature's source of the vitamin. As an orthopaedic surgeon, I deal with bone disorders daily and have long been interested in this topic. Because everyone in our sun-averse society is somewhat low in D_3, I just give supplementation then test them in a year after they have stabilized their levels. My vegetarian patients are the only ones I have routinely tested beforehand—just to prove to them how deficient they were. Carnosine (an amino acid) and DHA (an omega-3 fat found only in meats and fish) are also deficient in vegans and vegetarians.[10]

Perhaps most important, vegetarians are short of cholesterol in a usable form. Although cholesterol has gotten a bad rap over the years—more about this later in the chapter—it is critical to most body functions. Specifically, it is crucial to brain mass and brain function because neurotransmitters are made from cholesterol. It is also the precursor to sex hormones and adrenal hormones. Testosterone and cognitive (brain) function are both diminished in vegetarians and vegans.[11] Maybe this loss of testosterone explains why most of my vegetarian and vegan patients are women!

It is well worth reading *The Vegetarian Myth* by a former committed self-proclaimed vegetarian, Lierre Keith. In this well-written and very thorough book, Keith tells her story of being ill and depressed for more than twenty years until she finally could not resist the facts and started eating a diet that included meat. She addresses each argument in favor of a vegetarian lifestyle, including the argument from ecology. For the ecological vegetarians, she points out that returning to the more pastoral mixed agriculture of centuries ago is much more ecologically sound than the monoculture of today that produces the millions of acres of wheat and corn necessary for vegetarianism.

Keith has great sympathy for those who, like my patient, don't like to kill animals, but points out gently that they are not really keeping death out of the animal world by living a sickly, vegetarian existence. "The vegetarian ethic is still ultimately a variation on the mechanistic model. It simply extends our morality, whether humanist or religious, to a few animals that are similar to us. The rest of the world—the living, sentient, communicating agents who make oxygen and soil, rain and biomass—those billions of creatures don't count. . . . Their ethic is still part of the paradigm that's destroying the world."[12] As a sarcastic friend of mine has opined, most vegans' protective umbrella for animals really only extends to fluffy, furry animals with sad eyes—animals that can be anthropomorphized. They couldn't care less if a cockroach or sewer rat gets exterminated, and they probably swat mosquitoes without thinking.

THE STANDARD WESTERN DIET IS BAD IN A DIFFERENT WAY

It has been known for nearly a century that the standard Western diet produces health problems. In the 1920s Weston A. Price, a dentist and founder of what became the research arm of the American Dental Association, traveled the world, studying aboriginal cultures and the impact of diet on teeth and facial bone formation. In the process he came to believe that not just teeth, but general human health was adversely affected by a Western diet. He noted specifically that peoples as varied as the Maori and isolated Swiss villagers, while eating their traditional diets, had broader faces with straight teeth free of cavities. And they were also healthier in many ways, having less deformity, less tuberculosis, and fewer other diseases of modern civilization. When Dr. Price analyzed the foods eaten by these isolated natives, he discovered they contained at least four times the calcium and other minerals and ten times the fat-soluble vitamins from animal-rich foods. For the rest of his life, he promoted "real food for real people"—the idea that human-processed foods were to be eschewed in favor of natural, aboriginal-type diets including good, natural animal fats.

Others have written along these lines, including Gary Taubes in his book *Good Calories, Bad Calories*. Taubes notes that in Africa, before the introduction of the Western diet, diseases of modern civilization (heart disease, diabetes, and cancer) were rare. His excellent book, which focuses on obesity and the cycle of disease, reveals that diseases of modern civilization show up in an aboriginal culture, on average, seventeen years after the introduction of a Western diet. He ascribes the ill effects to four foods—white processed flour, white rice, sugar, and beer.[13] (Like it or not, he is probably right. Regarding the last one, note that we don't talk about martini gut, just "beer gut.")

Since the time of Weston A. Price, in spite of various food fads and the nonsense propagated by outmoded "official" food agencies, we have been drilling down closer to the truth. Recently, Dr. David Perlmutter, a neurologist, published *Grain Brain*, and Dr. William Davis, a cardiologist, published *Wheat Belly*, probably two of the most eye-opening and best books on the issue. In short, the major culprit in the Western diet responsible for the majority of the problems we see today is wheat or wheat gluten—a major staple estimated to comprise nearly 75 percent of the average American's intake.

WHAT'S WRONG WITH WHEAT?

"What's wrong with wheat?" you ask. Well, in a nutshell, everything. Wheat (after digestion) is the only food to cross the blood-brain barrier and bind with opiate (morphine-like) receptors. Wonder why you have food cravings? Wheat is an addictive substance. It gives you a craving to eat constantly. And it is an unnatural substance that we were not genetically designed to ingest and metabolize. Besides being nutrient poor in its own right, it has the unusual property of damaging the tight junctions between cells in the gut, thereby disturbing the body's ability to properly absorb nutrients from other foods. This effect is most obvious in people with so-called celiac disease, who develop overt diarrhea with wheat. But to a certain degree, many if not most people have a degree of digestive disruption.

And wheat in its modern form contains a substance called amylopectin-A, which produces autoimmune disease. Want to get rid of psoriasis? Stop eating all wheat. Stop wheat and stop the progression of rheumatoid arthritis and lupus. Now, you cannot just go halfway on this one. To be effective you have to eliminate all wheat from your diet, and I mean *all wheat*. It is not dose related, per se. Wheat is an immune trigger. Imagine turning on a football stadium's vast lighting with a single switch. A *small* switch—the trigger—can produce the *big result* of bright lights all over the stadium. So too, wheat is a trigger. Eating even a morsel can, in people with autoimmune disease, trigger a reaction in our immune system that lasts for months. I have had several patients with Crohn's disease (a problem that includes bloody diarrhea, gastric pain, and ultimately poor health from malabsorption of nutrients). The gastroenterologists—specialists in gut disorders—do not know what causes Crohn's disease, but they will swear that diet makes no difference. I am an orthopaedic surgeon. I do not pretend to be a gastrointestinal specialist. But I take health histories, and knowing what I know, I tell my patients about the emerging science of wheat/gluten sensitivity. In one case, an old friend from high school told me about his twenty-four-year-old son. This young man had developed all the symptoms of Crohn's disease—weight loss, bloody stools, diarrhea after eating, and abdominal pain. In general he just felt bad, with loss of energy and vitality. I told his dad, "Try taking him completely off wheat. What have you got to lose?" At the time his son was on about seven hundred dollars a month of IV medications, which, in spite of the high price, had failed to relieve his symptoms very much. Within three days of going wheat-free, however, all his symptoms resolved. Three days! I helped him wean slowly off his medication just in case symptoms would recur. But they never did. He remains well and committed to a strict wheat-free diet. As further confirmation of the cause of his problem—diagnosed by gastrointestinal (GI) docs as classic Crohn's disease—he accidentally ingested some wheat months later, and for a day or so the symptoms returned, including diarrhea. As of this writing, he has been asymptomatic for a year. Now, I call that a test of the theory. But sadly, his GI doctors still say diet doesn't matter. And in a self-fulfilling prophecy, they say if it was solved with diet, then it couldn't have been Crohn's disease.

What?! Well, I have two other such patients, and with time, perhaps others will believe in the wheat connection. And in time, after much needless patient suffering, the truth will out, as they say.

So, in addition to the addictive factor (gluteomorphine) and the autoimmune factor (amylopectin-A), modern wheat contains a big, fluffy starch that spikes your insulin. As noted before but is worth repeating, insulin is a fat-storage hormone. The caveman, who ate very few carbohydrates, had chronically low insulin. He was a lean, mean, hunting machine. In our wheat- and carb-saturated society, we constantly elevate our insulin, and this is responsible for our diseases of aging—especially obesity and diabetes. It is not fat that makes you fat. It is carbohydrates, and the worst of the worst is wheat.

I stopped eating wheat Christmas Day 2012. By June 2013, without really changing my exercise routine, I had gone from a size 12 to a size 6, had lost all the so-called cellulite from my thighs, and had reacquainted myself with the waist I had as a young girl. I also noticed that the loose stools I routinely had after eating my meals (this developed in my fifties) totally stopped. Wow, did my life change—with one simple dietary shift!

In his book *Grain Brain*, neurologist David Perlmutter reviews the world literature on wheat and brain function. Although doctors traditionally saw celiac disease as a gastrointestinal problem, it turns out the major organ affected may be the brain. Perlmutter provides ample citation about this widespread neurological disease due to wheat gluten, and how he has cured, or at least significantly improved, everything from ADHD to schizophrenia to depression—simply by cleaning up the diet and eliminating wheat. The new MRI technology has shown many headache sufferers to have an abnormal signal in the brain, and both the signal and the headaches go away when patients go off wheat. It was my fondness for an intact brain and clear thinking that finally pushed me to go gluten-free years ago.

SURVIVING THE MEDICAL MELTDOWN

WATCH THOSE OILS!

Another agribusiness-produced death factor in our Western diet is vegetable oil. Primitive man got fat from animals and perhaps from some olive, palm, and coconut trees. He did not squeeze a hundred acres of corn to produce Mazola. He did not eat Crisco or soy oil or canola oil or margarine. These vegetable (omega-6) oils produce inflammation in the body and are associated with arterial clogging. They damage not only your blood vessels but your brain, which is made nearly entirely of fat. Eat artificial oils, have an artificial brain. In this case, it may seem too simple, but it is that simple. The only oils that should cross your lips are olive oil, meat fat and lard, butter, fish oil, coconut oil, and palm oil. As an aside, it turns out that coconut oil is nearly perfect food for the brain, bypassing the metabolic block in dementia. Adding coconut oil to the diet of Alzheimer's patients has been shown in some cases to rapidly improve mentation. Recently Dr. Brian Peskin, a very smart and innovative researcher, has shown that PEOs (parent essential oils) are better at reducing vascular aging than fish oil (EPA/DHA). This is new information, but his studies done on patients by monitoring finger blood vessels are quite persuasive. His book *PEO Solution*, cowritten with Dr. Robert J. Rowen, is worth reading, and I expect their conclusions to be confirmed independently. His oils are available on the Internet.[14]

THOSE NASTY LITTLE EXCITOTOXINS

Another product of a Western diet is our exposure to *excitotoxins*, chemicals that are damaging to nerve cells by producing overstimulation of the cells. These damaging chemicals have crept into our food supply in boxes and jars and cans. You really don't get exposure to them if you "shop the circle"—eat foods from the outside circle of the grocery store (where all the fresh foods are) and avoid the inside aisles (filled with packaged pseudofoods). The big three excitotoxins are MSG, aspartame, and Tylenol. Yes, Tylenol. In addition to liver failure—where the science is quite well worked out—Tylenol is bad for the brain and the kidneys.

More than fifteen years ago, an article was published in the journal *Neurology*, looking at the risk of Alzheimer's in people taking anti-inflammatories. Anti-inflammatories include drugs such as Motrin, Advil, Naprosyn, Celebrex, Voltaren (Diclofenac), and Mobic. Whereas Tylenol is just a pain reliever, these anti-inflammatories block a chemical pathway that first and foremost inhibits inflammation; then, by this effect, they secondarily relieve pain. It was found in the *Neurology* study that those who took an anti-inflammatory medication for two years had a lower relative risk of Alzheimer's dementia, by about 50 percent, as compared to those people who took nothing.[15] This makes sense with what we know about Alzheimer's being partly an inflammation of the brain. In the main section of the paper, the data also showed that people who took Tylenol for two years *increased* their risk of developing Alzheimer's by 40 percent. Interestingly, this finding—buried as it was deep in the body of the study—was not reported in the news release or mentioned in the abstract summary of the article. (Increased Christmas bonuses to the Tylenol PR people!) So most physicians have not heard of this troubling information.

The mechanism for this brain injury is not yet proven, but it is thought to involve Tylenol's interaction with the NMDA receptor in brain cells. The NMDA receptor regulates calcium channels that lead to excitation of nerve cells, and this excitotoxicity is probably one of the final common pathways for the development of Alzheimer's.

In 1971 scientists reported on the appearance of brain plaques resembling the plaques in Alzheimer's that appeared after exposure to phenacetin—an older Tylenol-type compound.[16] Later, lending further credence to this concern, there have been reports of acute memory loss in patients with only ten days' exposure to Tylenol. When this Tylenol-induced memory loss happened recently to an oncologist, the doctor became aware of the same phenomenon in his patients, and he now is attempting to bring this to the attention of the medical establishment.[17] Fortunately, these acute memory losses seem to be reversible once the Tylenol has been removed. But memory is difficult to quantify precisely, so I don't think we can be sure of this.

Tylenol in the presence of alcohol poses a double whammy to the liver. Alcohol consumption decreases glutathione in the liver— a potent detoxifying agent for Tylenol. Combining alcohol with Tylenol can prove fatal even though the amount of Tylenol ingested is within the recommended dose limits. This is magnified if the patient has been fasting, which further depletes glutathione. Since 6 to 7 percent of Americans are heavy drinkers, and 39.5 percent of people between the ages of 18 and 25 report binge drinking,[18] and since the difference between the safe range and the unsafe range for Tylenol is relatively small, this makes the population very much at risk for adverse effects. Fasting—which may be involuntary after, say, surgery, also makes the liver more vulnerable to these effects. So having too much to drink, forgetting to eat or vomiting, followed by some Tylenol for hangover, is the "perfect storm" of toxic cocktail to the liver. There are numerous cases of acute liver toxicity and death from exactly this scenario.

Additionally, in a meta-analysis done at Harvard, prolonged use of Tylenol was associated with an increased risk of renal cancer (up to 33 percent), whereas aspirin and other anti-inflammatories have been shown to slightly decrease cancer risks.

Take a close look through your medicine cabinet. First look for all the obvious Tylenol medications—Tylenol, Tylenol PM, Tylenol Cough and Cold, and acetaminophen (the generic name for Tylenol). Next, look for any prescription pain medications you may have, such as Lortab or hydrocodone/APAP (the APAP means Tylenol has been added). Check cold medications—Nyquil, Alka-Seltzer Plus, St. Joseph Aspirin-Free, Zicam, etc. Any drug that has *APAP*, *cet*, or *acetam* as part of the name probably contains Tylenol. Notice how many of your medications contain acetaminophen/ Tylenol. This hunt is not just an academic exercise. The Tylenol people have done a great job of slipping their product into a myriad of commonly used drugs.

Instead of Lortab or other combination painkillers, I routinely give my patients plain codeine after surgery, but until I specifically asked for it, my local pharmacy had no common prescription narcotic painkiller without Tylenol. Generally, pain medicine given post-op contains Tylenol.

I never prescribe Tylenol for my patients. I warn my arthritis patients against any prolonged use, and I don't use it for myself and my family. Although all drugs have side effects, some effects are easier to deal with than others. The major side effects of anti-inflammatories are gastrointestinal ulceration and/or bleeding and occasional decreased kidney function with prolonged use. But kidney function is much more easily monitored than memory, which may be gone before the patient realizes the problem. And this type of kidney function is generally reversible. For now, I would expunge Tylenol from your medicine cabinet. If you are going to have surgery, talk to your doctor about a pain reliever that does not contain acetaminophen. And if you must take a Tylenol-containing medicine, be sure to supplement with N-acetyl cysteine, which boosts protective glutathione in the liver.

Aspartame is the sweetener in our diet soda drinks, although some manufacturers are beginning to use sucralose and even stevia, a totally organic plant leaf–derived sweetener. The dangers of aspartame are debated, but biochemically it acts like an excitotoxin, displacing the ion channel blocker at the NMDA receptor. Knowing the physiology, I'm not waiting for a thirty-year study to tell me definitively it is bad. I stopped drinking all diet sodas the day I was attending an "anti-aging" seminar, and the lecturer caught me drinking a Diet Pepsi and said, "You actually still drink that stuff?" It is generally believed in that crowd that aspartame is the work of the devil. When I quit drinking the diet sodas, I got a headache that was variably present for three months—and I never get headaches. I thought the headache was due to caffeine withdrawal, but subsequently I have drunk and stopped drinking caffeine in a form that does not contain aspartame, and I did not experience a prolonged headache. Although this is not a rigorous study, I believe that aspartame is an independent risk factor for headache and withdrawal from such drinks. It is most probably an excitotoxin and bad for the brain.

THE HIGH FRUCTOSE PROBLEM

Finally, don't expose yourself to a darling of Western agribusiness—high fructose corn syrup. Regardless of the corn processors' PR campaign, the truth is, high fructose corn syrup causes liver dysfunction and obesity. I have seen patients with elevated liver enzymes, who were extensively studied (to include liver biopsy) without coming to an understanding of their problem. When the patients eliminated all high fructose corn syrup from their diet—presto! The liver functions normalized. Again, I don't have thirty-year studies to prove it, but it doesn't take too many of these observations to make one a believer in the liver-altering power of corn syrup.

And in spite of the protests of the corn syrup producers, high fructose corn syrup *does contribute* to obesity. Here is how it works: You have a very sophisticated hormone system—the leptin–ghrelin system—that controls weight by controlling appetite and other factors, but appetite is the most important issue for the purposes of discussing corn syrup. In the old days—let's go back to the 1950s—when a teenager drank a Coca-Cola from those old, greenish glass bottles, he was taking in about 100 calories of real sugar. His body sensed these calories via the leptin–ghrelin hormone system and diminished the kid's appetite proportionally. So for dinner, instead of eating 759 calories, his appetite cut off at 659. He lost out on 100 calories of real nutrition to ingest 100 calories of sugar, but at least he didn't overindulge.

But here is the rub. High fructose corn syrup is a new product interacting with an age-old genetic makeup. And the leptin–ghrelin system simply doesn't see it, so it doesn't count this 100 calories of high fructose corn syrup when calculating the body's appetite suppression. So now the kid goes ahead and eats his full dinner, not having any dampening down in his appetite. And if he drinks more than just one cola with high fructose corn syrup with his dinner, many calories can slip by unnoticed by his innate appetite control system. It's the perfect formula for obesity. And sadly, schools, instead of employing real cooks and serving home-cooked food made from real ingredients, have opted for prepackaged crapola from various national food services. One of my favorite anecdotes about school food was told to me by my younger son when he was a freshman in high school. He attended a mandatory assembly at which time they were forced to watch the movie *Super Size Me*—a very interesting documentary of a man who purposely ate every meal at McDonald's for an entire month. The movie is worthwhile because there are actually some very interesting points made, including the fact that it was better financially and much better nutritionally if schools went back to having home cooking by real cooks, rather than the prepackaged, Sodexho Marriott stuff. At the assembly, the movie was paused midway, and the kids were let go for lunch—to go eat Sodexho Marriott prepackaged artificial crap. So apparently, this mandatory assembly was not about science or nutrition but gave English credits for "irony"?

THE CHOLESTEROL AND LOW-FAT MYTH

There has been no more pernicious and persistent lie perpetrated upon the American people than the idea that to be healthy we should eat low fat and specifically avoid cholesterol. During the time we have been following that advice, we as a nation have become sicker, fatter, and more demented. Great. And now we are doubling down on this bad idea by lowering cholesterol levels even further using "statin" drugs. Unfortunately, this is a prime example of business, rather than clean science, driving medicine. Although it is true that anyone can be wrong, that even the best minds err, and we in medicine have not always treated disease properly, when we err—in the absence of compelling economic interest—the error is usually short-lived. It is only when billions of dollars are riding on a medical treatment that truly bad ideas can be promulgated widely, scientific dissenters quieted, cheering sections bought, and the truth suppressed for decades.

Funding flows to those whose ideas reinforce the consensus opinion—right or wrong. So, although we have known for decades that ingested cholesterol does not per se raise blood levels, business has too much money riding on low-cholesterol foods to admit that fact. Additionally, we know that lowering cholesterol has not diminished mortality from heart disease. It has changed the pattern of disease but has not lowered overall mortality. Although per-haps—and this is still a perhaps—statin drugs (the most common cholesterol-lowering medicines) have decreased heart attack rates slightly, death from heart failure has gone up. And there is good physiology to explain this effect, adding credence to the point. We also know that many people who experience heart attacks have cholesterol in the normal range.

The fact is, cholesterol is extremely important not only because your brain is made of it but also because it is converted to neu-rotransmitters and—as I said earlier—sex hormones. The idea that low cholesterol is desirable and improves longevity is not true. Lowering changes the pattern of disease. We know that "oxidized" cholesterol—in other words, damaged cholesterol—is bad. But in the absence of damage through oxidation to the cholesterol particles circulating in the blood, it appears that higher levels of serum cho-lesterol are better in many ways. The biggest issue is what cholesterol does for the brain. The Framingham study of diet shows that choles-terol levels were proportionally related to verbal fluency, attention, reasoning, and other cognitive outcomes. People with cholesterol above 240 did better than people whose cholesterol was below 200.[19]

According to Dr. Perlmutter in his excellent book *Grain Brain*, the *Journal of Alzheimer's Disease* recently published research from Mayo Clinic on older people, their diet, and their brain function. The study found that people whose diet was highest in good fats had 42 percent less chance of cognitive impairment; in other words, brain dysfunction.[20] And I remember him saying at a lecture I attended that people who for some reason had very high levels genetically, in the 350 or higher range, *never* got Alzheimer's—or at least he had never seen it happen in those patients. Butter does not seem to benefit the brain (although it does not appear to harm it), but fish oil, olive oil, flaxseed oil, and walnut oil were beneficial. And coconut oil is very good. Parkinson's disease is also related to low cholesterol.[21]

SO WHAT SHOULD I EAT?

It is impossible for me to summarize all the studies and footnote all the recommendations I am making. I designed this eating regimen based on a lifetime of interest in the subject, combined with a sophisticated medical education and a recent fellowship in integrative and complementary medicine through the American Academy of Anti-Aging Medicine. In the reference section you will find books that are highly footnoted that go over the science in grim detail—some of which we have discussed in this chapter. But you have the power of common-sense observation, so I challenge you to just look around at the people you know and what they eat.

In a nutshell, the caveman and you were meant to be meat eaters, eating a diet consisting of meat with its fat, nuts, berries, and vegetables. To quote my hero, the late Jack LaLanne, "If man made it, don't eat it." Here are my guidelines for an optimal diet:[22]

1. Start with a low-carb diet. If possible, 10 percent or less of your calories should come from carbohydrates. At least keep carbs below 30 percent, but shoot for the lowest you can manage.

2. Eliminate all forms of wheat.

3. Limit milk to one cup daily, but yogurt, cheese, and other forms of milk products are good.

4. Do not eat "low-fat" anything. Low-fat products contain thickening agents that are the worst forms of carbohydrates. Eat full-fat milk, full-fat yogurt, etc.

5. The only oils that should cross your lips are the naturally occurring omega-3 oils: meat fat, butter, olive oil, coconut oil, palm oil, and fish oils (or PEOs). I allow myself occasional mayonnaise, which does contain soy oil. I have discovered that in eating man-made foods, it is best to pick brands that have been around for decades rather than new products. The older ones have better and simpler ingredients. Add a little coconut oil daily to your diet. I either put a dollop of it on a cracker, or I make a dessert using full-fat coconut milk as outlined in *Grain Brain*.

6. When eating meat, it may be best to eat grass-fed meat or wild game, but that is not always possible or financially feasible. I try to make up the deficiency in grain-fed beef by supplementing with conjugated linoleic acid (CLA). Eat chicken without hormones, and limit cured meats. Organ meats are especially nutritious and healthy.

7. Fish is great, but there are several things to keep in mind. First, bottom-feeding fish and shellfish may collect heavy metals, so they shouldn't be a huge part of your diet. Second, farm-raised fish does not contain natural goodies such as omega-3 fats and also may have heavy metals due to the runoff from the land into the fish beds. In general, a varied diet avoids over-accumulation of toxins and heavy metals.

8. Eggs are nearly perfect human food. If you can raise your own chickens, do so—it's a lot of fun and produces the very best eggs you will ever eat. If not, get home-raised eggs from your neighbor. If you can't do either of those, try to get omega-3 eggs or eggs from free-range chickens.

9.   Eat lots of cruciferous vegetables—broccoli, cauliflower, Brussels sprouts, cabbage, kale, etc. Vegetables, in general, should fill the part of your plate not filled with meat and fat. Although most vegetables are healthiest with the least amount of cooking, it turns out that tomatoes actually become better with canning and cooking. The nutrients in them become more available to the body with processing.

10. Modern fruits are hybridized to have too much sugar. So generally, the best fruits are berries or low-sugar fruits, such as old-time apples (like Winesap, Jonathan, or Alexander), pomegranates, kiwis, etc. The idea of eating five servings of fruits (or whatever the latest mainstream mantra is) is patently wrong. It will add weight. Nutritionally, you will do much better eating vegetables.

11. Nuts are a good snack—specifically walnuts, pecans, almonds, and Macadamia nuts. Peanuts are not as good but can be eaten in small amounts.

12. Drink fresh, clear water. Get off all soda pop. Recently, a University of Iowa study linked diet soda consumption to increased cardiac death in women. While this may be just a marker for an unhealthy lifestyle, all the cola drinks have something bad in them. Also, I actually don't think a power drink in the morning in lieu of coffee for a little caffeine boost is bad. These drinks have sucralose and no phosphoric acid (which is bad for bone), and they add taurine (an essential amino acid) as well as other nutrients. I would limit them to one or two a day, however. One of the best drinks for a little flavor is green tea. Green tea is an antioxidant and anticancer drink. It has been shown to work better on prostate cancer than some cancer treatments. Also, it is associated with improved weight loss in people on diets.

13. The question always arises, "Should I eat organic foods?" In my opinion, "Organic" is a label that has lost quite a bit of meaning. If it really meant that organic foods were grown without using chemicals and had a really low

level of toxins, then maybe. But the definition has been morphed by agribusiness and politics, and it is almost unintelligible. For the small-potential but ill-defined benefit, you will pay a high premium. I don't pay it. I try to grow as much as I can in my own garden, buy good-quality food, and wash things carefully before eating. I avoid additives and GMO (genetically modified) foods as much as possible. There is a great deal of controversy about GMO foods. I didn't used to be concerned about GMO foods, but my personal experience with gluten has opened my eyes to the possibility that a genetically modified food may contain harmful and unique substances in proportions not present in the ancient parent plants. The foods my pioneer ancestors ate were very different from the foods most of us eat today. For example, modern hybrid apples feed our cravings for sugar and carbohydrates. Probably one of the hardest addictions to overcome is our addiction to sugar. It seems we have an inborn desire for that sweet taste—probably as an adaptation for foraging. Even bacteria will swim upstream in a sugar gradient to get more sweetness, and they can't be accused of having a "sweet tooth." So it is not surprising that we humans have modified our foods to satisfy inborn cravings.

In sum, health is 90 percent diet related. Past generations suffered from scarcity of food, but the food they did eat was *real* and compatible with the human body's genetic blueprint. There is much evidence that the diseases of modern civilization—diabetes, stroke, heart disease, and cancer—are in large part due to our diet. And it is not just overeating. It is eating substances that look like food but in reality are like Frankenstein—artificial, manmade, and unholy creations that even bacteria will avoid. If we are to optimize our health and lifespan, we need to consciously reestablish the eating patterns of our ancestors. We need to literally "feed our genes" what they were meant to have—nutritious, natural, clean foods using the guidelines above.

9

PREPARING YOURSELF: EXERCISE

There is a general misperception that exercise is the key to losing weight and that to be effective, exercise must be vigorous and/or extreme. But exercise is not the key to losing weight. Although the more muscle you have, the more calories you burn and the easier it is to *maintain* weight, the compelling reason to exercise is to optimize fitness for the future.

I once read an ex-Soviet discussing America. He said that if America were to have an economic collapse similar to Russia's after the fall of the Soviet Union, Americans would not fare well. Russians were accustomed to foraging for necessities even in good times—normally walking miles a day. In contrast, Americans were so out of shape they would be unable to survive this and would "blow out" their knees. He is probably right. Just sit in a public place and count how many healthy and fit-appearing people pass by—very few. In fact, recently I made a similar observation at a Walmart where I was sipping ice tea and waiting for a friend.

Exercise does two very important things. The first, improving your cardiovascular fitness, is what most people associate with exercise. The second, and intimately related, is that it increases strength. In the world of tomorrow, I anticipate more need for manual labor.

We may need to grow our own food, carry things without as many gasoline-powered automobiles to help, and build things without the power we are accustomed to. I hope I am wrong, but if I'm right, this will require functional fitness—that is, strength and coordination. And this means muscle.

There is a funny ad that is supposed to promote a chain of fitness centers. The small, thin, male representative is escorting a huge, bulked-up bodybuilder through the facility. At each "station," when the fitness center representative tries to describe the workout machine, the weight lifter just keeps saying in his thick Nordic accent, "I lift things up and put them down." He is summarily escorted out the back into the alley. The fittest people are not welcome, I guess.

But if you want to improve your heart fitness you need to lift. If you want to improve your stamina, you need to lift. If you want to improve your bone quality, you need to lift. We are meant to be muscled. Cardiac fitness is not an end to itself. When you lift weights, your heart gets stronger and your vessels better support your basic human function, which is to move and to lift and carry. When you use your muscles to near their capacity, they get stronger, and they improve the cardiac system to support the activity. I know you have been told you have to run a lot to do "aerobic conditioning," but it is not true. You can lower your resting heart rate, you can get lean, and you can improve your body's oxygen carrying capacity by lifting. And along the way, you keep your weight in a good range because muscle is the driver of metabolic rate. The runner burns a lot of calories during running, but the rest of the time does not burn the calories a guy with lots of muscle burns. The weight lifter burns more calories all the time. If you really want to decide for yourself the best form of exercise, just do what I have done and make a study of people in the gym. You should not use college gyms as a measure, because young people have not yet hit the problem of midlife fitness. But look at a public gym—I use Anytime Fitness because they are really "anytime" and pretty much anywhere. Look at the people using the "cardio" equipment—the elliptical, the stationary bicycles, the treadmills—these are the "cardio bunnies." There is usually a row of fattish bodies jiggling like crazy on those machines. Then look over at the weight lifting area. It is rare to see anyone with excess fat. These people, the ones who pick up heavy things and put heavy things down, range from slender and defined to very muscular, but rarely fat.

Now, it is okay to do some running or cycling or tennis or whatever you like. But if you want functional good health, focus on weights and hit the running trail for twenty to thirty minutes three times a week. Short-duration, high-intensity aerobic exercise complements weight training.

I lift weights but do not pretend to be an expert on training weight lifters. The general thinking of today's lifters is to focus on compound lifts, not small, single-muscle repetitions. For beginners I refer you to an excellent book by Mark Rippetoe, *Starting Strength: Basic Barbell Training*. It is simple to use and understand, and it explains the correct way to do compound lifts for functional weight training. It is far less helpful to do a bunch of barbell curls than it is to do a standing dead lift or a bent-over row. Compound lifting not only builds muscle in the extremities but also creates trunk strength and coordination. This is why Midwest farm boys have traditionally been such champion wrestlers—because baling hay produces more overall functional strength than isolated individual muscle exercises in a gym.

The other important principle to understand is that the body never stagnates. It either builds muscle or stores fat—it never pauses in between. And this happens on a day-to-day basis. If you exercise today, your body (whose genes go back in time at least to Cro-Magnon hunter-gatherers) thinks it is hunting, that there is food on the Serengeti, and that it needs to build muscle to chase the antelope. On a day you sit with a book all day, not doing much, your body thinks it is in a cave, that food is scarce, and that it needs to survive until there is food available. So it stores fat and/or chews up muscle for energy. Although oversimplified, our metabolism is somewhat like a two-position switch, which is either growth or decay.

The truth about exercise is very simple: you should move and you should lift things. If you do that at least thirty minutes a day, you will maintain adequate fitness. The more you do, the fitter you will become—to a point. This new extreme-sport lifestyle is often counterproductive. Women who exercise to the point of extreme thinness are not helping their long-term overall health. While they may have aerobic capacity, they have lost their body fat and therefore their estrogen storage capacity. This leads to infertility, thinning of bone, and other metabolic problems. Men who run marathons or do extreme cycling or any exercise that results in a slightly cadaveric appearance, are not really helping their health. Extreme exercise that breaks down a lot of tissue creates too many toxins in the body and destroys muscle. It may make people feel some psychological boost from the achievement, but it is not a longevity or wellness prescription.

I lift weights three days a week for thirty minutes to an hour on average. On another three days I either do a twenty-minute run down and up a steep hill (to work crosswords at the local Chat 'n Chew) or run intervals for thirty minutes on a treadmill when it is icy or too cold. I take one to two days off. And if I take an extra day off, it is from running—not the weight program.

A good way to gauge your fitness is to check your resting pulse in bed as soon as you open your eyes. Adults (children normally have faster rates) who are in poor condition often have resting heart rates over eighty-five beats per minute. Well-conditioned people will have resting pulses of around sixty or even slightly less.

Another way to check for cardiovascular fitness is to note how long it takes for your pulse to return to normal after exercise. If you are still tired and have an elevated pulse thirty minutes after stopping your exercise, then you have some conditioning work to do.

In sum, strength is king. Complex exercise is better for strength and coordination. Aerobic conditioning should be done in moderation, and interval training is better than long, slow distances, which do not facilitate muscle gain.

10

PREPARING YOURSELF: SLEEP

In chapter 8, we dealt with a natural diet, the diet the caveman would have eaten. Similarly, sleeping should mimic the caveman's habits. In her excellent book *Lights Out*, T. S. Wiley outlines the hazards of electric lights and artificially prolonging our days. We were meant to sleep with the sun cycle. When the sun comes up, you start the day. When it gets dark, you go to sleep.

This natural sleep cycle is important for health and longevity. It has been shown that disruption of animals' circadian rhythms shortens their life span. Humans are cyclic animals. We live by sun and moon.

Women's fertility in a natural state is timed to the moon cycle—ovulation occurring around the time of the full moon. Our sex hormones—testosterone, estrogen, and others—as well as our adrenal and thyroid and growth hormones are produced in response to cycles of day and night and to light from the moon cycle. As humans have adopted modernity, living in artificial electric light has changed our natural rhythms. By artificially extending our days, we are sacrificing our hormonal rhythms. For example, it has been shown that just applying a light to the back of the knee in a dark room can shut off hormone production.

In studying patients' hormones I have noted that adrenal function was normal only in my farmer patients . . . even though they were in their seventies and eighties. They generally lived by the sun cycle. Conversely, my young doctors and nurses, with totally abnormal schedules, were all adrenally insufficient to the degree that their sleep was disrupted.

When I was doing trauma surgery I was frequently awakened in the middle of the night or would spend the whole night in the operating room. Although at thirty this didn't seem like such a problem, by the time I was fifty, it was a big problem. I couldn't get to sleep without reading for hours, and at two to three in the morning, I would awaken and not get back to sleep for another few hours. I felt more and more dreadful as I became more sleep deprived. After starting a full anti-aging program of hormone replacement, exercise, and supplements (including supplements for sleep, described later in the chapter), I was better. But laboratory testing still showed my adrenal function to be flatlined, and usually I still was not sleeping well through the night. My stamina was still down. For this and other reasons, I sold my big solo practice, quit my trauma call, and moved back to my rural roots. After two years of sleeping in a quiet bedroom that faced a dark, forested backyard, I was much better. I chose a bedroom in the house that faced away from all streetlights so the only light entering my bedroom at night was the moonlight. I slept with no curtains, and during the full moon I noticed that I did not sleep as soundly. But I accepted that as part of normalizing my hormonal cycle. Now I still take sleep supplements, but I sleep through the night. My adrenal function is significantly better on lab testing. I feel great and awake refreshed—not drugged out or dragging. But it didn't happen overnight. It took years and patience to overcome many years of bad sleep. I took melatonin on faith for three months before I realized that I was falling asleep more easily. Then little by little the corrective measures paid off.

As we get older, our sleep often becomes more and more difficult. Here are the major culprits, but I'm sure there are others:

1. Artificially extending the day with electric lights.

2. Caffeine. Caffeine can build up. What you can tolerate at twenty-five may not be tolerable at fifty-five.

3. Noise. Noise can come in a variety of forms, from the street noise to a spouse's snoring.

4. Hormone problems. Hot flashes can be very disruptive of sleep, and although primarily a woman's issue, it can actually affect men if they lose their testosterone rapidly.

5. Loss of brain transmitters and hormones with aging and disease (melatonin and serotonin being the most important for sleep).

6. Deconditioning.

7. Anxiety.

8. Medications.

It is not always possible to find *one problem* that is the issue. Although you may have an idea what is causing your sleeplessness, you really should run the list and correct everything that might be a culprit. Begin with good "sleep hygiene." As noted earlier, sleep with the sun cycle, and avoid extending your day with electric lights. Suzanne Somers, in her excellent talks on wellness, tells of her evening ritual. When it starts to be dusk, she dims her lights and may add candles. You should also get rid of TVs, radios, and computers in the bedroom.

If there is a noise problem, consider a pink noise generator to block annoying sounds. (Pink noise is simply white noise with the harsher tones removed.) Unfortunately, one of the very common noise problems is a snoring spouse. It may be God's little joke, or maybe it is for child rearing, but the fact is, women sleep less soundly than men. And men are overrepresented in the population with sleep apnea—often characterized by loud snoring. If your partner is filling the room with loud snoring and you are tossing and turning, then you may need to sleep in a separate room while you are convincing him to get evaluated. (The snoring in sleep apnea is due to upper airway obstruction from the tongue or soft tissues in the oropharynx. Sleep apnea is a major cause for sudden nighttime death and heart attack due to oxygen levels falling from the obstruction.)

Wean yourself off all caffeine. Caffeine is often used to get started in the morning because you feel sleepy. But it becomes a positive feedback loop. The more you juice yourself to get going in the a.m., the worse you sleep in the p.m.; then you up the dose of caffeine. Once you are caffeine-free and sleeping well, however, you can try adding it back in the early morning a little at a time. I do find a little caffeine helps sport performance, but it can easily get out of hand.

Consider bioidentical hormone replacement if hot flashes are disrupting your sleep. This is discussed at length in a later chapter, but trust me: hormone supplementation works to improve sleep and generally to make you feel better.

If you have difficulty getting to sleep, try melatonin sublingually (under the tongue). As we age, melatonin production goes down, and it is the hormone that gets you to sleep. Melatonin not only helps you get to sleep but is also an anticancer hormone. So, there are many reasons to take melatonin. It must be sublingual to have the best sleep-inducing effect. Begin with 3 milligrams at night. I would not increase the dose for a month. After a month, if you still need more than thirty minutes to get to sleep, double the dose to 6 milligrams under the tongue at night, and continue to do this until you have no difficulty falling asleep. Generally, no more than 12 milligrams under the tongue should be required. A sign of having too much melatonin is having very vivid, unpleasant dreams. I once dreamt that my husband turned into a big green lizard and slithered out the end of the bed. That is typical of melatonin-induced nightmares, which tend to have a very bizarre, surreal quality. I find that sometimes I need more melatonin than other times. When I have taken on too many projects and my mind is running away with me, or on Sunday nights—probably because I have to get up especially early to drive eighty-two miles to my job—I take an extra pill under the tongue.

If you can get to sleep but cannot stay asleep, or have early-morning awakening, you can benefit from taking 5-HTP at bedtime. This drug produces serotonin, a neurotransmitter that helps one stay asleep. For this reason it should be taken with caution by people on antidepressant medications (SSRIs) that inhibit the reuptake of serotonin. It is good to understand your medications and discuss this with your doctor before starting this over-the-counter pill. For most people, though, I would start with 25 to 50 milligrams at night. This can be swallowed or taken under the tongue. Again, I would not up the dose for a month unless it fails to give you the required result. Then I would double the dose to up to100 milligrams. If you're still having morning or midnight awakening, then you might consider taking another 50 milligrams at noon.

Loss of the American electrical grid would be an unmitigated disaster. We would lose critical manufacturing, critical drug production, and more. I can think of only one good thing to come out of an economic crisis or other problem that would shut down the electrical grid for a prolonged period—we might get back to nature and sleep better. But we can voluntarily take steps to re-create nature, and that is clearly the better alternative. So as T. S. Wiley exhorts, "Lights out!"

11

PREPARING YOURSELF: SUPPLEMENTS

For years physicians have been saying that "vitamins just make expensive urine." That statement is cute, but it is simply not true. Recently the news reported studies presumably showing a deleterious effect of fish oil. And almost like a Greek chorus, the medical community was quoted as saying, "There is no evidence that supplements are beneficial."

This is clear nonsense, and doctors know it—they take supplements themselves. And for their patients, they know that vitamin C supplements prevent or treat scurvy. They give vitamin B_{12} shots to patients with pernicious anemia, and they advised the milk industry to add vitamin D to prevent childhood rickets. This is "supplementation." What they are really saying is—they don't want you to make your own decision to supplement your diet in the absence of their medical input. But as I have pointed out previously, scientific advances are slow to percolate into the actual practice of medicine. So, even if it were proven beneficial to significantly elevate blood levels of vitamin D (as it has been), it would take decades for the medical establishment to be fully on board.

As a consequence of individual genetics, diminishing capacity to absorb nutrients as we age, and eating a generally poor American diet, many people develop deficits of certain nutrients over a lifetime. These nutrients are involved as "cofactors" in chemical reactions that convert food to energy, detoxify, support cell growth, and provide immunity. Our understanding of these processes over the last thirty years has expanded tremendously, and now we can test for very specific deficiencies of these vitamin cofactors. Then we can tailor supplements to the individual.

Let's start with a quick review of biochemistry. We will use as an example the process of methylation, which is an important function for many body processes. Vitamin B_{12} is a cofactor in the methylation process, which moderates and inhibits the expression of certain genes. B_{12} works together with an enzyme to help regulate gene function.

There are important genetic differences in people's ability to methylate because of the activity of the enzyme. This important chemical activity is enhanced by elevating the level of the cofactor, vitamin B_{12}. A one-size-fits-all mentality is incorrect in medicine in general, but particularly when looking at levels of cofactors. I may be able to methylate with a little B_{12}, and you may need five times as much. Therefore, measuring B_{12} levels is inadequate. We need to measure some aspect of the ongoing chemical reactions to check if they are proceeding as needed. Fortunately for B_{12}, there is a cheap test that does just that. A reaction that involves methylation is the conversion of homocysteine to methionine. By measuring the level of homocysteine (and there are others), we can determine whether methylation is occurring appropriately.

Today, there are a myriad of such processes we can measure. It is possible and not overly costly to test the effectiveness of the chemical processes that convert food to energy, and then to correct for deficiencies. Organized medicine recognizes so-called inborn errors of metabolism, but only the most overt ones. Practitioners of standard medicine willfully ignore the possibility of less profound—but deleterious—individual genetic variation of everyday metabolism. And in spite of many studies showing benefits of various supplements, they continue to chant, "Supplements don't work."

Even without specific testing, it is known that Americans generally are deficient in certain cofactors. The supplements I recommend to everyone are chosen because they compensate for our unnatural dietary patterns. For example, fish oil (or probably PEOs, as mentioned earlier) is needed to compensate for the fact that the aboriginal human ate fish and grass-fed wild game, so they naturally had a high intake of omega-3 versus omega-6 oils. Traditional hunter-gatherer diets contained about a 1:1 ration of omega-3 to omega-6. Today's grain-fed beef and farm-raised fish simply do not give us the same quantity of omega-3 fat as wild game did. And vegetable oils are high in omega-6. These oils are not naturally occurring. It took the advent of modern agribusiness to efficiently squeeze corn to make corn oil—primitive man's arteries were never exposed to the stuff. Beginning at the turn of the twentieth century the consumption of these man-made oils as well the introduction of feedlots and processed foods have dramatically changed the oil ratio. Estimates vary, but it is reported that by 1900 the ratio of omega-6 to omega-3 was 4:1, and now it's about 25:1.

OIL	OMEGA-6 CONTENT	OMEGA-3 CONTENT[1]
SAFFLOWER	75%	0%
SUNFLOWER	65%	0%
CORN	54%	0%
COTTONSEED	50%	0%
SESAME	42%	0%
PEANUT	32%	0%
SOYBEAN	51%	7%
CANOLA	20%	9%
WALNUT	52%	10%
FLAXSEED	14%	57%
FISH	0%	100%

This has dire consequences for the arterial wall. Dr. Barry Sears has written *The Anti-Inflammation Zone* outlining the need for omega-3 oil in various medical conditions.[2] I asked him personally about the amount needed for healthy people, and he suggested 3 grams a day. It is important not to take in rancid oil. Oil should be kept cool and not kept over a few months. If it smells rancid it is not good. For this reason I do not use the cheap oils from big box stores, but I buy mine from places that keep the oils chilled or sell in bulk frequently. Life Extension Foundation at www.LEF.org is a good source. I have transitioned into using PEOs. (See chapter 8 for more information about oils and PEOs.) And of course, I eat a low omega-6 diet. The point is to have a normal blood ratio.

IODINE

Another dietary problem in modern society is our lack of iodine and our increased intake of bromine (as outlined in chapter 8). Everyone in America needs iodine supplementation because we do not eat like the Japanese who ingest hundreds of times more iodine in seaweed. Iodine is critical to thyroid health and is probably an anticancer element. Most iodine in stores is very low dose, on the order of 150 mcg (micrograms), whereas the Japanese ingest 12.5 mg (milligrams). I order "Iodoral" 12.5 mg on line—there are various sources, but as far as I know this is the only brand available in a large enough dose to make a difference.

ZINC

In my experience testing a number of people with advanced tests, nearly everyone—even children—is deficient in zinc. Zinc is critical in intercellular signaling, and it facilitates skin healing. It is a component in most of the OTC cold remedies because it seems to help the body respond to invading viruses. I suspect our soils have been leeched out of this mineral. But for whatever reason, we need to take at least 7 mg if not 15 mg a day. Plastic surgeons give 220 mg a day for a few days to help wound healing.

MAGNESIUM

After observing elderly people in the hospital, I have realized we have a tendency to have lower magnesium with age. And by the time it is low in the blood, it is very low in the cells because the body will leech out the magnesium from cells to preserve blood levels. Our deficiency is probably due again to our diet, which tends to be repetitive and not as natural as it once was. Low magnesium is associated with hypertension (high blood pressure) and headaches. If you don't have hypertension or headaches, I recommend everyone take 400 mg a day of magnesium. If you have hypertension, you may benefit from much larger doses. My former anti-aging nurse got off her blood pressure pills by taking 1,200 mg a day of a slow-release magnesium.

VITAMIN D

Everyone is low on vitamin D—even people who work and play outside. Instead of wasting a patient's time and money with testing, I simply recommend some supplements. If there is one anti-aging hormone (D is not really a vitamin), it is vitamin D3. (See the paper on vitamin D in appendix A.) I recommend 10,000 units a day for people without renal problems. No one has overdosed on that dose, and it is less than an aboriginal will get in nature when living on the equator.

Without specific testing, I recommend the following for everyone (if you have certain medical conditions, such as renal failure, you must consult a physician first):

SUPPLEMENT	DOSE	BENEFIT
FISH OIL OR PEO	3 G OR 1,500 MD/DAY	VASCULAR HEALTH AND ANTI-INFLAMMATION
IODORAL	12.5 MG/DAY	THYROID FUNCTION / ANTICANCER
MAGNESIUM CITRATE OR MALATE	400 TO 1,200 MG/DAY	BLOOD PRESSURE CONTROL, BONE HEALTH
SUBLINGUAL B12 WITH FOLATE	1,000 MCG/DAY	NERVE HEALTH, BLOOD FORMATION
VITAMIN C	1,000 MG/DAY	IMMUNE HEALTH
VITAMIN D3	10,000 IU/DAY	NEARLY EVERYTHING
ZINC	7 TO 15 MG/DAY	IMMUNE HEALTH, SKIN HEALING

In short, there is a scientific basis for taking supplements. Life Extension Foundation (www.LEF.org) offers a very extensive summary of literature supporting specific supplements, and their reviews of the science are easy to read and accessible to people without medical backgrounds. Other references are *Dr. Blaylock's Wellness Report* newsletter or the American Academy of Anti-Aging Medicine at www.worldhealth.net.

12

PREPARING YOURSELF: HORMONE REPLACEMENT

Hormone replacement is perhaps an unusual topic for a survival book. But as it turns out, hormones are critical to health. Classic medicine—for some reason unknown to me—has approached the topic of hormones in a strange and ostrich-like fashion. Although most doctors measure and treat thyroid hormone problems, they have assiduously avoided dealing with adrenal hormones (except in the most severely deficient cases) or the sex hormones—testosterone, estrogen, progesterone. And don't even mention "growth hormone," or you'll have to call the special agents from the DEA.

Classical medicine spends huge amounts of time and money measuring things like potassium and glucose and magnesium levels. But these are the *downstream products* of metabolic activity. The *controllers* of metabolic activity in the body are the hormones—and we ignore them. It's stupid, and medicine is slowly starting to change. But you shouldn't wait thirty years until we get smarter or at least more informed. As I say in my lecture on anti-aging medicine, "Don't wait until you are dead."

OVERVIEW

Here's the big picture according to everything I have put together over a lifetime of studying physiology and, recently, anti-aging science. Our bodies are made up of many, many cells. Each cell maintains itself and contributes to some bigger overall function. To do that, each cell must be able convert digested food to energy and then use the energy for its specialized activity. If the cell is a muscle cell, the energy goes to producing more muscle protein and for causing the muscle to contract and relax. If it is a skin cell, it produces keratin to reinforce the skin. A stomach lining cell produces digestive acid, and so forth. The nucleus of each cell is a protein factory. This nuclear factory contains the blueprint for the entire body in the form of DNA. As we eat food, the cell turns it into energy and into the building blocks to make new parts for the body. The cell takes the amino acids that came in as our food, and it shuttles them to the nucleus, where they are recombined into new proteins using the DNA blueprint. These proteins are then incorporated into the body. In short, your cells are constantly producing proteins that become you.

All this protein building takes energy, so within each cell are little furnace organelles called the *mitochondria*. These mitochondria produce all the energy required for the body to move, breathe, and run its chemical reactions.

All these processes take place under a generalized scheme, which is not entirely understood. The ultimate conductor of the body's functions may not yet be known, but we do know that hormones are the major cellular level controllers. Take for example the mitochondrial energy machines. Thyroid hormone is produced in the thyroid gland in the neck. The thyroid gland takes protein and iodine and selenium and other substrates and combines them into thyroid hormone. This circulates around in the blood, and depending on what's happening to the body, it becomes more or less active. Then it attaches to every cell receptor and sends signals to the mitochondria to crank up the energy production. People without enough thyroid hormone get cold, lose hair, and gain weight because metabolic activity decreases—in short they become slugs. People with too much hormone start getting very warm and hyperactive, and can develop rapid heart rate, excessive weight loss, and sweating. Most people do not exist at either extreme, but in a fairly normal range of thyroid function.

Now let's consider the other hormones: adrenal hormones act on the cells to produce a variety of products that give us stamina and allow us to deal with stress; sex hormones give us our appearance, help maintain our weight, influence energy, and alter our sex drive; insulin tells cells to store fat; other hormones influence appetite. It goes on and on. But here is the point: there is no biologic advantage in losing your hormones. When we start to feel the effects of aging in our forties, it is due to a noticeable decline in our hormone levels. If hormone levels are not normalized by supplementation, then our cells are not getting the correct controlling signals. Our cell nuclear factories then start putting out abnormal proteins, and those abnormal proteins are incorporated into our bodies. We start feeling older and generally less vital after forty because we are slowly being replaced, protein by protein, with a new, abnormal us.

THE CANCER SCARE

In addition to good diet, adequate sleep, and a sound exercise program, I recommend, and I myself use, hormone supplementation. Women have used hormone therapy for years, but recently concerns about hormones raising cancer risk were voiced after early results from the Women's Health Initiative were poorly communicated to the public.

The concerns about cancer were overblown from the get-go. In short, the Women's Health Initiative is a long-term study looking at a variety of health data. It was gleaned from the data that women on postmenopausal hormone therapy had a very small increased rate of cancer. But it turns out the conclusions were very misleading and essentially wrong. When the results were more closely examined, it became apparent that the small bump in cancer was completely attributable to use of an artificial chemical called *progestin*. It is not correct to equate progestin with natural progesterone. Progestin is a man-made pseudo-hormone whose function and life cycle in the body are very different from the natural hormone progesterone. Because it is disposed of differently, progestin goes through a fairly toxic phase before being eliminated from the body. The carcinogenicity of progestin was again confirmed in recent studies in Europe, where large groups of women on various postmenopausal regimens were examined, but *the only group* to have increased cancer rates was the group taking progestin. Having said all this, even the increased cancer rates reported were offset by the benefit to women by lowering mortality from heart disease.

Suzanne Somers is a breast cancer survivor, and she is currently taking the same Wiley hormone replacement I use. Before starting that program I contacted the cancer specialist following her and about fifty others on the Wiley program who also have had breast cancer. As it turns out, although this data is unpublished to my knowledge, the rate of cancer recurrence in the treated group was far below the rate of recurrence in people not on the program. For my money this makes sense because one of the many benefits of hormone replacement is an improvement in immune function.

BIOIDENTICAL HORMONE THERAPY (BHT)

For women this is somewhat complicated because normally we have hormones that wax and wane with the moon cycle. Men are simpler and have less cyclic variation and fewer hormones to worry about. For men, replacing testosterone to normal ranges is usually all that is required; albeit some men, like women, need thyroid and adrenal assistance. Generally, oral therapy would not be used for sex hormones because of its effect on the liver. So we use patches or rub-on creams or injections. For most men, I find a simple rub-on cream dispensed via a pump is fine. They push the pump and it gives a measured dose, which they rub on some part of the body that won't come into contact with other people. (Women partners don't need much testosterone and can get overdosed from a man if he does not take precautions: wash hands, use under clothing when going to work, and avoid the buttocks, where it can transfer via toilet seat.)

In my female program I replace thyroid and adrenal hormones orally and then use rub-on creams to replace estrogen, progesterone, and testosterone. There are several things that all anti-aging doctors agree on: (1) these hormones do not cause cancer, (2) there is no anti-aging benefit to being without hormones, and (3) oral sex hormones are bad. But we do not all agree on the way to dose and monitor hormone supplementation. There are those who give women the lowest dose possible to prevent symptoms such as hot flashes. Then there are those who give a higher, steady state dose. And finally, there are those who replicate the hormone levels of youth by giving high-dose hormones cyclically. For myself I use the higher-dose cycling hormones—I re-create the environment for my cells that I had in my youth. I very much believe the philosophy of T. S. Wiley in her book *Sex, Lies, and Menopause*, that our bodies were made to cycle. And in addition to the voluminous literature debunking the idea that cancer is produced from bioidentical hormones, I try to think about this logically. Who gets cancer? Women in their twenties whose estrogen and other hormones are sky-high? Or women in their fifties with declining hormones in abnormal proportions? We know the answer is the latter. In my own experience, I feel the best, look good, and have normal menstrual cycles when using the cycling youthful level of hormones. At sixty-one I actually feel better and am in better shape than when I was forty-five. And whereas I once hated having my menstrual period, now I celebrate the monthly blood flow as biofeedback that my cells are normal again!

To get on a program of hormone optimization, you will need to find a doctor or nurse practitioner who specializes in this field of medicine. You may find one by word of mouth or the Internet. But if needed, I have listed resources for finding a practitioner.

PART III
LIVING THROUGH THE MELTDOWN

13

BE YOUR OWN CORPSMAN:
INTRODUCTION TO PERSONAL SURVIVAL

Having been a Navy medical officer for ten years, I have a great affinity for Navy corpsmen. At the battle of Iwo Jima, Navy corpsmen and surgeons landed with and were everywhere tending to wounded Marines. After that historic fight, four Congressional Medals of Honor were awarded to Navy corpsmen, two posthumously. John Bradley, one of the flag raisers at Mount Suribachi, was, in fact, a Navy corpsman. In Vietnam, 620 Navy corpsmen were killed, more than three thousand were injured, and four corpsmen earned the Congressional Medal of Honor.

Independent duty corpsmen, or IDCs, are the highest level of medical care aboard many submarines and surface ships. They also supply medical care for the forward-based Navy and Marine Corps Special Forces teams. Through multiple conflicts, on land and on sea, in remote areas, in inclement regions, clever Navy corpsmen have learned how to survive and how to medically assist those around them—often with little in the way of supplies or oversight. We have much to learn from their experience, so I am using them as a model of independent medical care when higher-level medical help is either absent or far away.

INFORMATION IS KEY

Because the future is always uncertain and you never know what medical crisis may come your way—or if help will be help available in such a crisis—it is probably a good idea to get a military field medical reference, such as the *Special Operations Forces Reference Manual* (see appendix A). It is wise to print out pertinent sections to keep in case of emergency. I'm not confident about our ability to have complete access to the Internet in the future, so I keep very important information backed up by paper. Also, a plethora of self-help, home-care manuals are available at major bookstores. Some may be better than others, but definitely purchase something and keep it handy. As much as I disagree politically with the AMA, they put out a great home book for emergency care, the *American Medical Association Handbook of First Aid and Emergency Care.* The more portable, the better. The U.S. Army *First Aid Manual* is an excellent small book of the nuts and bolts of first aid care that can easily fit into a backpack or your seventy-two-hour bag. This book is intended to be a quick reference for many things. For in-depth assistance, the *American College of Physicians Complete Home Medical Guide* gets high praise from laypeople for its thoroughness, good illustrations, and general helpfulness in understanding all sorts of diseases.

BUDDY CARE

One of the principles of military medicine is buddy care. It is important that family members be organized and that everyone understand how to help others in certain emergencies. If one family member has periodic, severe asthma attacks, all able members should be trained to assist if needed, including knowing where important medicines are stocked. Everyone should take a CPR course and should understand basic first aid. All the principles of evacuation and emergency meeting areas should be part of a family's planning.

ORGANIZING SUPPLIES

Navy corpsmen know that it's prudent to distribute supplies among many users. Of course, in a combat situation this is done for many reasons, not the least of which is to camouflage the corpsman, who otherwise is one of the prime targets. But it is also done so that no one ends up carrying too much and so that if one bag gets left behind or lost, you are not totally without medicine and supplies.

Most survival handbooks recommend that every family member be responsible for a pack. From a medical perspective, this pack should carry that person's prescription meds, over-the-counter meds, and supplements for at least a week. You can possibly replace food and water, but you may not be able to quickly make up prescription meds.

I also recommend having a more extensive first aid pack that can be hand carried. In that pack I would put basic supplies, splints, and more medications. Suggested contents are outlined in appendix B.

And it is probably a good idea to have a true first aid emergency backpack for grab-and-go. There are few areas of America without some realistic disaster potential that might necessitate emergency evacuation—forest fires, tornados, floods, earthquakes, to name a few. And then there are gas leaks, toxic spills, and industrial accidents. Don't be complacent about organizing for an eventuality you hope never occurs.

Being a physician, I have organized my packs around specific problems. You could use various-sized backpacks or plastic storage boxes for your packs. I have one box of wound care supplies; another for advanced wound care that includes minor surgery sets; one box for respiratory problems; one for medications; and my father's black bag, which contains examination equipment—a stethoscope, some old-fashioned mercury thermometers and a new one that does not require a battery, a blood pressure cuff, and so forth. I also have several boxes of supplements and hormones. Finally, I have a pack of splints, slings, and orthopaedic equipment that I keep—for obvious reasons—next to my snowboard bag. I have a second, tiny house that is my peripheral office. It is eighty miles away, and I keep there a seventy-two-hour medical kit. If for some reason I had to bolt out of my regular home, I would go with my family there. It is probably a good idea to distribute survival medical supplies among family members' seventy-two-hour kits, and each member should carry a kit. In the military, corpsmen do carry some things, but every ground combat unit distributes medical supplies among *all* its members.

COMMUNITY SUPPORT

Consider, too, that in an emergency, most of your neighbors will be less prepared than you. I have participated in a group that has given preparedness talks to our community because we do not want to be surrounded by desperate, unprepared people. Consider organizing your community for a general catastrophe, and then get a medical provider to help with this piece of the preparation.

It is the principle of the Mormon Church and of the Jews at Passover (and probably at other times) to prepare for one's own family plus one other person. I would think that way about supplies in general. When it comes to medical preparedness, depending on the catastrophe, you may want or need to render first aid to others. The level of preparation depends on how you see your role in this eventuality. As a surgeon, I am now the repository of all out-of-date wound care articles from my hospital. I am preparing to be the community medical clinic in a pinch.

In the next few chapters, I will outline in detail what to stock in your packs, but the first thing you need to know is where real emergency and nonemergency medical care can be found. That's what we'll discuss next.

14

FINDING A PHYSICIAN WHEN PHYSICIANS ARE SCARCE

Years ago, I read an article in the *American Journal of Medicine* that said that 90 percent of the time people go to a doctor, they don't really need a doctor. But that other 10 percent of the time, they need a damn good doctor. I believe that to be true. Of course, the key is knowing whether you are in the 90 percent or the 10 percent. A good Navy corpsman knows where his resources are for that 10 percent.

It will become important for you to have a relationship with some higher-level medical provider—a physician, nurse practitioner, nurse, or physician's assistant. You need to assess the resources you have and keep that information updated and handy. Think of it as you would your will and testament. You try to keep a list of people who need to be contacted for quick access by your heirs. Of course, the best insurance is to do what I did: I sent my son to medical school! (Actually he went of his own volition in spite of my telling him to be a lawyer.) But since everyone can't do that, you need a list of all medical personnel you can access in an emergency.

As stated in previous chapters, those people most likely to be left out in the cold in the coming medical meltdown are those of or near Medicare age, the disabled, and those with chronic disease or potentially terminal illness, such as prostate cancer or myeloma, with which you may live for many years but whose treatment may be deemed "futile."

Ultimately, if things become as grave as I believe they will, we will all be in trouble finding the medical care we need, either because an economic collapse impacts our ability to trade goods and services—including medical care—or because there simply won't be a doctor or a clinic for miles and miles.

As an aside, but in confirmation of this fear, I recently attended a mandatory training session for EPIC. EPIC is the most common electronic medical records (EMR) system being forced upon hospitals and physicians' offices. Nothing in my career has proven so devastating to quality health care as the implementation of EMR. As it turns out, the CEO of EPIC was a huge financial backer of Obama—big surprise? But the upshot is this: all four of us at the training were surgeons in different specialties and from different hospitals, and we all discussed how we could retire rather than deal with this awful nightmare.

I am going to assume that the government in this scenario has not made cash payment for medical care illegal. If, however, the government outlaws cash practice (as was done in Cuba, Canada, the Soviet Union, and North Korea), then most of this chapter still applies to getting care in the black-market economy that will surely develop.

FIND A CASH PHYSICIAN

Most doctors today don't work for you—they ultimately work for those who pay them—in other words, insurance companies and the government, via Medicare and Medicaid. Having said that, it is also true that most physicians are true professionals, and they do try to keep your needs at the forefront of their consideration. But ultimately, let's face it—they run a business, and if they lose money on a treatment, they can't continue to offer you that service. (This is a basic business concept that seems not to be understood by policy makers in DC). And when the system collapses, those dependent on government fees being paid by Medicare will collapse with it and not be available—at least for a while—to help you.

Thankfully, a growing number of physicians are running cash practices. They do not take any government money, so they don't have to follow government rules and are not dependent on a functioning government system to stay in business. Because a cash practice requires far less staff, their overhead is low. They are usually very cost-effective, charging a fraction of what is charged through insurance. And in any case, they spend time with you, not with your records, so you get more for your money.

There are several ways to employ a physician for cash. The easiest is to find a physician who is already set up to accept cash. There are three groups of these physicians: (1) conventional physicians who have "opted out" of the system and have strictly cash practices; (2) anti-aging physicians (also known as "integrative" or "complementary" physicians, who generally only work for cash; and (3) concierge physicians—think the TV show *Royal Pains*, about catering to the rich in the Hamptons. Not all concierge physicians are so highbrow. Many are affordable to middle-class people who want to prioritize health over other expenditures, such as the latest Ski-Doo.

CONVENTIONAL CASH PAY PRACTICE

If you are sick and need routine care, or if you are strapped for cash, you might seek out a conventional cash pay practice. Many of these can be found by calling around to physicians in your local area. But there are also resources such as the Association of American Physicians and Surgeons—an organization that promotes cash medicine (AAPSonline.org). For the names of cash physicians in your area, go to aaps.wufoo.com/reports/m5p6z0/. Other options are SimpleCare (SimpleCare.com), MediBid (Medibid.com), and DocCost (DocCost.com). At the time I began this book, these cash-only physicians were few and far between. But in the last year, with the nightmare of EMR and Obamacare, more and more docs are opting off the government plantation and opening cash practices. An added benefit to all cash practices—whether they are doctors or PAs or nurse practitioners—is privacy. They won't be sending your most intimate medical information to bureaucrats in the federal government or to your insurance company.

ANTI-AGING PHYSICIANS

If you are well and have a little more money to spend, it may be best to seek out an anti-aging physician. The two big educational players in the field are Cenegenics and the American Academy of Anti-Aging Physicians. They both have websites to help you locate their physicians. The American Academy physicians are listed on WorldHealth.net, and Cenegenics-trained physicians can be found at Cenegenics.com. These doctors hold standard medical licenses but have joined the rapidly expanding group of physicians offering complementary or integrative medicine. Traditional government-compliant medicine demands strict adherence to conventional wisdom as revealed in the standard medical literature and teaching. This results in medical care that is out of date by the time it hits the paper or the government-approved algorithm, and you, the patient, receive medical care that is often twenty years out of date. In contrast, anti-aging, integrative physicians incorporate the latest science and clinical observation into their thinking. (See chapter 3, "Why Your Doctor Is Out of Date," to understand this in more detail.) These are the guys who help you not get sick—as opposed to just bailing you out once you do! The downside is, many of these doctors do not want to be your "primary" physician but would rather just work on the wellness aspect of your health. I believe, however, that as things collapse, they will take on more and more of their patients' needs.

FIVE THINGS TO LOOK FOR IN CHOOSING AN ANTI-AGING PHYSICIAN

1. Do they recommend supplements?

2. Do they balance all your hormones, not just the thyroid?

3. Have they completed or are they pursuing postgraduate training in "anti-aging" or "integrative" or "complementary" medicine?

4. Do they allot at least an hour for the initial visit?

5. Do they do nutritional counseling?

WHAT TO AVOID IN CHOOSING AN ANTI-AGING DOCTOR:

1. Ask if they use bioidentical hormones. If not, keep looking.

2. Avoid university- or hospital-based or government-run health clinics. Look for independent, usually solo, cash physicians.

3. Since physicians right out of residency have not been trained in anti-aging thinking, it's best to find someone at least five years or more out in practice.

4. Avoid physicians who do not appear healthy themselves. Is the doctor obese? Is he or she a smoker? You wouldn't hire a home builder who lives in a falling-down shack; why trust a physician who is not following a healthy lifestyle?

CONCIERGE PHYSICIANS

"Concierge" physicians cater to high-end clients. If you can afford this level of "Cadillac" care, you are in good shape. They take cash. They usually practice high-quality medicine, and some, but not all, practice avant-garde anti-aging medicine. And they become your primary physician. You can access information about them by going to their association website, http://www.aapp.org/. A link to the list of their member physicians is on their home page.

Judging physician quality is complicated. Some of the flashiest fast-talkers, with the best bedside manner, may not be up to date or, as they say, "the brightest bulb in the box." On the other hand, I have known brilliant doctors and outstanding surgeons who were lousy in communicating with their patients. Just keep in mind the difference. It's a problem of style and substance.

When choosing a concierge physician, you use the same criteria as you do for other physicians: look for someone who meets your needs and knows about your problem or what you want to accomplish, and ask around. How do that physician's patients feel about him or her? Do you have friends who are nurses or doctors? What do they think? Even checking with others can be a problem. Every study looking at quality outcomes and patient satisfaction has shown that patient satisfaction is negatively related to quality outcome. In other words the worst outcomes were associated with better impressions of their doctors. It is unclear why this is true, but physicians are not there to be your friend, and "tough love"—insisting that you eat right, take medications, exercise, and so on—may not be as well received as the advice from a doctor who liberally hands out narcotic pain medications and tells you your health problem is not your fault.

Ultimately, you don't know a physician until you try him or her out. With concierge medicine where a regular fee is required, make sure there is an exit clause. If you don't like or trust the doctor, how does the contract get canceled?

All such care is threatened by the expansion of government medicine—in particular, Obamacare. Because people are not signing up in numbers to keep the program afloat, it is likely the government will use its eight-hundred-pound executive order sledgehammer and squash cash practices. They will do this by forcing all doctors into the government system. You the patient will probably not see this coming, as it will be done outside of Congress through administrative regulations. The Department of Health and Human Services will most likely inform states that to keep their federal medical funding, they must insist that all physicians accept Medicare and Medicaid. The minute they do that, the small cash practices (which have run at low overhead and low patient cost) will not be able to function. They will have to hire office staff and add administrative suites and a computer system to bill the government. Then they will no longer be what you wanted when you sought them out—they will no longer be able to offer medicine that is independent, state-of-the-art, cost-effective, and personal.

FOUR THINGS TO KNOW ABOUT CONCIERGE PHYSICIANS

1. Concierge physicians cost a premium but give premium service, including twenty-four-hour access.

2. Some, but not all, concierge physicians are "integrative" or "anti-aging" physicians.

3. Concierge physicians tend to be located in bigger cities.

4. All concierge physicians take a direct, regular fee from patients for their premium service, but most then charge your insurance as well when care is rendered.

STANDARD PHYSICIANS

If none of these options is available, you may be able to negotiate cash prices with your current physician or another one in your area. At present, physicians are allowed to work for cash *if* the patient is not eligible for a government program (such as Medicare, Medicaid, or Tricare) and *if* the patient is not signed with an insurance program with which the doctor is contracted. In other words, if you are now on Medicare, you have lost the right to contract privately with a physician unless that physician has formally "opted out" of the Medicare system. If you are legally able to pay cash, *do not accept the standard fees.* Standard fees are set to compensate for the enormous hassle of paperwork and waiting months to years to get paid by third parties. When you pay cash, the doctor gets a big break and should be able to pass this off to you. But you may have to convince him. Also, unless he has formally opted out from Medicare, he cannot legally charge you less than Medicare-allowable rates, even if you are not of Medicare age.

DOC IN A BOX

Go to many malls or Walmart–type stores and you will see cash clinics run by doctors or nurse practitioners. These offer low-level care for many routine matters, and they are cost-effective. In our Obamacare environment, these "Doc in a Box" shops are becoming more appealing to physicians and patients. They are not generally for long-term care of chronic illness; but for those who are generally well, they provide the kind of care the old-time country docs did—no frills or fancy testing, but quick fixes for many problems. In some of these shops, by charging cash at the time of service, they avoid all the hassles of inefficient electronic medical records mandated by the government. They can provide good quality for cost because they don't have to factor in the cost of complicated billing (estimated at fifty-eight dollars a bill). And they are not hindered by the thousands and thousands of pages of Medicare and Obamacare regulations, which demand—among other things—data collection on aspects of a person's life and health that are completely extraneous to the matter at hand.

HIRE YOUR OWN DOCTOR

Rich people have always had the means to hire their own "private" physician. But why not extend this concept to a group of average people? Let's say there are no cash doctors in a town of a thousand people. As the system collapses, patients have to travel farther and farther for care, and ultimately it becomes unavailable. If each of these people chipped in two hundred dollars and were then willing to pay a small fee per visit, the group could have a private physician all to themselves. The physician, no longer under government pay and rules, could run an old-time, cost-effective office, and the people could have easy access to local care. I used dollar amounts in this scenario, but remember that in an economic collapse everyone is affected—doctors too. So these numbers are just hypothetical, based on today's going rates.

FIND MID-LEVEL PROVIDERS

There is no question that physicians—MDs and DOs—have much more training than the "mid-level providers"—nurse practitioners, nurse midwives, and physician's assistants. But for everyday care these mid-level guys are great. And in the current environment, where doctors are scarce, these providers are taking up a great deal of slack in rural areas, where people would otherwise have no care. It has been my observation that mid-levels find their niche, and they really perfect that niche. I worked for many years with a PA doing nothing but spine surgery. Besides bringing a great deal of maturity and life experience to the job—he used to set himself on fire daily as a welder before becoming a PA—he became an expert at diagnosing and outlining treatment for patients with spinal stenosis. He would frequently see patients who had been through four or five specialists with extensive and costly workup, only to figure out their problem in a few minutes of careful history and exam.

Of course, these mid-levels function best in an environment where they can get quick curbside consults, as needed, from physicians in the building or nearby, and that may not be possible in the future. Nevertheless, they generally are well trained, use good common sense, and have years of experience in some area of medical delivery. I routinely see a nurse practitioner for my yearly Pap smear and minor needs. Everything mentioned about cash practices and hiring a physician could be applied to these providers. Just like automobiles or violins, they cost less and you get less (in this case, knowledge and technical training), but then again, how many of us buy a Bugatti to get us from point A to point B when we can buy a very nice, cheaper Nissan that gets the job done?

PROCEDURE	DOCTOR	FNP	PA	MIDWIFE
ROUTINE EXAM	X	X	X	
ORDER LABS	X	X	X	X
SEW WOUNDS	X	SOME	X	
SURGERY	X			
DELIVER BABY	X			X
HYPERTENSION	X	X	X	
DIABETES	X	X	X	
CHF	X	SOME	SOME	
COPD	X	SOME	SOME	
CANCER	X			
FRACTURES	X		SOME	

Ultimately, there are people with some medical training who live near you. Get to know who they are—the emergency medical techs, the former military medics, the licensed practical nurses, and the registered nurses. Get to know your neighbors. Attend the fire and rescue charity event. Volunteer at the blood drive or the hospital. Anyone with some knowledge may be able to help in some circumstances. Before government became our safety net, our communities were our sources for help. They will be again. It is good to have a skill to trade for someone else's medical skill or some negotiable item to trade—currency or food or bullets. Who knows what it will be? But talk to those around you and learn where your resources are.

When the Supreme Court sold out liberty by accepting the

constitutionality of Obamacare, people all around the country contacted me for comment. In response, I sent out a picture of me in surgical scrubs, standing on the side of the road with my dad's old, black doctor's bag, holding a cardboard sign that read, "Will Do Surgery for Food." And it may come to that. I am stocking up a home office for the possibility.

PAYING FOR YOUR MEDICAL CARE

If you are not on government-funded health care, the most cost-effective solution is to sign on with a cash physician for your everyday needs, and pay cash. Then buy high-deductible catastrophic insurance for those times that you have a major medical issue, such as surgery, heart attack, or cancer. If you need to, ask your employer to give you the money in your paycheck that is being paid for insurance; then buy your own care. Note that I said "care," not "insurance." Yes, I hope you will purchase some form of insurance, but you have to start thinking of buying care. If you have learned nothing else so far in this book, you should have learned that insurance is not synonymous with care and insurance doesn't guarantee medical care. You will find you are financially ahead because group insurance is vastly more expensive than private insurance for generally healthy individuals. Unfortunately, as the result of Obamacare, even high-deductible insurance has become significantly more expensive. And the plans for this government-administered nightmare change daily, so I cannot be more specific.

If you are of Medicare age, you should still seek out a cash doctor because, in the future, your Medicare doctors may discharge you from their practice, or they simply may not have the resources to care for you. But, how do you afford essentially paying twice for your health care? Establish yourself with a cash doctor, and see that physician often enough so that he or she knows you and considers you one of the practice's regular patients. This may be twice yearly or yearly—depending on the physician's requirements. If you need treatment above and beyond that, you may be able save money by using your Medicare benefits—as long as they are available-—with another physician if testing or hospitalization is required. This may not be acceptable to your cash doctor, so you need to be careful how you handle the situation. Many Medicare patients always use the cash doctor because cash doctors generally spend more time with the patient. Although it costs more, the value per dollar is much higher.

Don't forget barter. My father opened his office the day the banks closed for the depression of 1929. Not infrequently he got paid in the currency of the local farmers: ducks, chickens, and hams. I have taken floor laying and Kansas City barbecue in exchange for medical care. In the old Soviet Union, medical care was bought with shoes, food, and any comestible the people could scrape together to bribe the doctors and nurses for medical care.

START NOW

Do not wait until care is unavailable. Start now by weaning yourself off the system. If you stay with what you have until it is unavailable, you will not be able to easily jump ship. And typically we always get sick at the most inopportune time. You want to develop a relationship with a freethinking, non-government-dependent physician *before* the system collapses.

15

BE YOUR OWN CORPSMAN: STORING AND STOCKPILING MEDICINES

E very independent adult has a medicine cabinet, and it seems to get bigger as we get older. This may be adequate for today's needs, but in the event of a medical meltdown, you will need an expanded, well-thought-out medicine cabinet—not just the little one behind the mirror in your bathroom. Included in the 90 percent of things you may be able to care for yourself are: common febrile illnesses, diarrheal diseases, minor scrapes and cuts, sinus infection, minor eye infections and scratches, sprains, arthritis pain, rashes, insect bites, contact allergies, simple broken bones and dislocations, neck and back pain, and external ear infections. To this end you will need a systematically stocked medicine cabinet. (Appendix B has a list of drugs and a table of disease-specific medicines.) There are various cost-effective ways to build this. You should check out farm animal supply stores for medical supplies.

The farm or vet store drugs are cheap, and the quality is good. The same drugs we use on humans are also used on animals. But because they do not have to undergo FDA testing for the animals, because they do not have to meet the same packaging requirements, and because they don't have to be dispensed by pharmacists, they are sometimes much cheaper—especially if bought in bulk. A cow does not have to sign a disclaimer at the checkout window that it is declining counseling about the side effects of the drug it is being given. Everything has a cost. And just like food, the requirements for purity *may* be less. But honestly, I have no qualms about using farm store drugs. (Although I cannot in my medical practice officially recommend the same, remember: we are stocking for the time when standard medicine may not be available.) I am reminded of a famous '60s drive-through fast-food joint in Nebraska. They were known for miles around for having excellent chili. Teenagers hung out there, and many people flocked there for this excellent chili. But the garbage man always wondered why there were so many Alpo cans in the trash every week. As it turned out, they were making their famous chili with Alpo—to save money and increase profit, of course. But the point is, until it came to light and violated a health ordinance, no one cared. Canned dog and cat foods have more contaminant parts per million and may not have the top-quality cuts ground into them. But they are nutritious, and I'd sure eat them before starving. So, too, with these medications. They are produced by the same companies, are packaged well, and are extremely unlikely to be significantly different from those given to humans. If you are in doubt, you can choose not to use them.

FARM STORE ANTIBIOTICS

Cipro and clindamycin used together are a great broad-spectrum (kills many types of germs) antibiotic combination that we use commonly for infections of skin and bone—especially puncture wounds.

Amoxicillin is a good start for ear infections that are internal, and it will work against strep throat. (Keep in mind that *most* sore throats are not strep but viral, and antibiotics do not work against viruses.)

Doxycycline is used for treatment of Lyme disease, for post-exposure prophylaxis, for urethritis (infection of the tube from the bladder), and for some sexually transmitted diseases. Regarding potential bioterrorism, all the drugs listed will treat anthrax. Doxycycline can also be used against plague and tularemia, also known as rabbit fever.

DRUG	FARM STORE	PHARMACY (CASH PRICE)
CIPRO	$0.84 PER TABLET	$19.59 FOR 20 CAPSULES
DOXYCYCLINE	$58.40 FOR A 30-DOSE BOTTLE	$124.73 FOR 30 TABLETS
CLINDAMYCIN	$1.26 PER 150 MG CAPSULE	$22.53 FOR 30 CAPSULES
AMOXICILLIN	$0.48 PER 500 MG CAPSULE	$22.20 FOR 30 TABLETS
CEPHALEXIN (KEFLEX)	$0.48 PER 500 MG CAPSULE	$19.23 FOR 30 CAPSULES

Certainly topical antibiotics are equivalent and effective. Also, most drugs do not become magically worthless at the "use by" date shown on the bottle. Ask most physicians. Since we cannot ethically write prescriptions for narcotic pain relievers for ourselves or our families, we hang onto any such medicine prescribed by the dentist or other physician so we may use these for injuries sustained years later. I learned the hard way to take a bottle of narcotic pain medicine with me along with basic slings and splints on all snowboarding trips. It cost me $750 just to have a retired cardiologist in a ski-slope clinic tell me—an orthopaedic surgeon—that I had a clavicle fracture. I needed the sling and the pain medicine, so I had to pay the price for information I really didn't need—having diagnosed my own fracture the minute I hit the icy ground!

Long-term expiration dates are extrapolated from short-term studies that subject medicines to temperature and light and other extremes that seldom replicate conditions in anyone's medicine cabinet. There is no literature—except in the case of a form of tetracycline no longer in use—that confirms that expired drugs cause harm. I don't worry about harm. I do worry a little about efficacy.

The one drug I know about that does degrade and should be replaced when expired is the epinephrine in EpiPens for allergic reactions, such as bee stings.

THREE THINGS TO KNOW ABOUT EXPIRATION DATES

1. Outdated drugs have not been shown to be harmful.

2. Most drugs retain their efficacy for years past the expiration date.

3. Never rely on outdated EpiPens; always keep these updated.

The Department of Defense, in conjunction with the FDA, has been testing for the loss of chemical stability of 122 medications for more than twenty years.[1] Two thousand six hundred fifty lots of drugs were kept unopened and left on a shelf. They looked at potency (chemical assay), physical appearance, water content, and dissolution. No chemical failures were recorded one year past expiration date. Four hundred seventy-nine lots failed after an average of sixty-five months. There were no failures of amoxicillin, cipro, or doxycycline, or of potassium iodide tablets (kept by some people for use in nuclear accident/radiation exposure).

Now, of course, these were unopened bottles on a shelf in moderate temperature and no light. It doesn't translate to a bottle of aspirin left in the back window of your car in Phoenix over the summer. But in general, I keep drugs for years. If they smell too much like vinegar (aspirin degrades to that smell) or are crumbling or don't look right in any way, I get rid of them. I don't automatically dispose of them when the expiration date comes. Keep in mind that expiration dates make money for pharmaceutical and other medical supply companies.

One time I was about to scrub up for a spinal surgery and found that all the Hibiclens surgical hand scrub had been removed from the sink dispensers. When I asked what had happened, I was told that cases of Hibiclens had "expired"—i.e., were older than the stated "use by" date on the bottle. This meant that the hospital disposed of cases of perfectly good soap to be replaced by more costly new soap. Why should Hibiclens hand soap expire? Does your home dish detergent expire? Some of this is clearly nonsense for profit. (I demanded that some outdated soap be used in the interim, pointing out that a surgeon not scrubbing before surgery was probably a bigger deal for sterility than Hibiclens that was a few weeks too old.)

STOCKPILING PRESCRIPTION DRUGS

Because shortages are sure to occur with the vast overregulation that Obamacare piled onto Medicare and OSHA and the FDA, you should stockpile at least three months and preferably six months of any medicine you need. This includes hormone replacement. When you fill your prescriptions, your insurance may pay for only a month or ninety days at a time, but *you can pay cash* and get more. Do it. You can often pay less for ninety days of a generic medicine than you would pay for just the co-pay of a name brand. For example, for ninety days of Singulair—a name-brand asthma medicine—I might pay a fifteen-dollar co-pay but at the cost of a much higher monthly premium. But for seventeen dollars with a much lower monthly premium, I can buy one month of montelukast, the generic equivalent, thus saving myself a couple hundred a month in premium costs. Also, insurance companies give you a little fudge factor on the amount you can get. They may authorize ninety days, but at the eighty-day or seventy-day mark, they will let you get another ninety days. So by being careful, you should be able to slowly add to your stocks.

Another option is to utilize an overseas pharmacy. Many winter visitors to cities along the Mexican border go across the line and purchase their prescription drugs for cash. The savings can be so significant that it pays for their winter vacation. On overseas trips

I have purchased antibiotics over the counter in India and in Italy. I am often asked about quality of these overseas pharmaceuticals. Again, I cannot officially recommend them in my role as a licensed US physician, but I can tell you that for me, I am willing to accept the uncertainty about quality (and there is always a degree of risk even for US medications) in return for ease of purchase and astonishingly lower prices. I want good packaging and usually try to get a brand with which I am familiar. In the 1980s, while I was on active duty in the Navy, I flew on Alitalia; and in those days, having observed the Italian telephone system, I was more worried about flying Italian airplanes than ingesting Italian medications. Every aspect of life has risk. In spite of our government doing its best to regulate each fragment of medical care in the name of safety, it is ultimately up to the individual to judge risk versus benefit.

To keep medications fresh, rotate the medicines so nothing outdates and always keep a stash to survive three to six months. Refrigerate when necessary. Again, as noted before, in modern history, when countries experience monetary collapse, it usually takes at least three months for the monetary system to be restored to a degree that allows goods and services to flow. You need to stock for this probability. And I am stocking for longer—under the assumption that when America goes down, it will shake the world more than the fall of Zimbabwe or Argentina.

Next, I would get some antibiotics—either via a friendly physician, buying them over the border, or via a farm animal supply. I keep antibiotics that cover most minor things and also most treatable bioweapons agents (see appendix B).

The government has made it hard for honest people to get and store some spare narcotics, but druggies seem to have no problem. As the government becomes more and more intrusive and oppressive and penalizes doctors for overprescribing, you will be less likely to get any surplus pain medicine from an injury or surgery or tooth problem. I would hoard what you can now. That's what I do. (Feds now are probably on their way to kick in my door.) Put those in the emergency first aid kit, and distribute any spare narcotics either to other adults' packs or into a special med pack. The important thing is not to let it get to children accidentally. (Although multivitamins with iron probably hurt more children than codeine does.)

CHILD SAFETY AND YOUR STOCKPILE

Of course, it is extremely important not to let small children access any medication or supplement. People generally hide or secure their prescription medications, but the sad fact is, multivitamins with iron historically have hurt more children than prescription medications because we don't recognize them as dangerous and therefore do not secure them from small hands. In 2011, according to SafeKids.org, 67,700 children were seen in emergency rooms for medicine poisoning.[2]

For our purposes, there are two parts to child safety and medications: storing our stockpile and safely maintaining those medications you use every day. For the stockpile, the safest option is storing it in a locked closet. However, not having one in my house, I keep my stockpile on a high shelf in an unlocked closet. The key is, it is well out of reach of toddlers and small children. For everyday medications this is not practical. If you use your medications from a medicine cabinet, purchase a locking one. People often keep their daily medications and vitamins in the kitchen for easy access. If you do that, I suggest a wall-mounted locking medicine shelf. Wayfair. com carries a thirteen-by-five-inch horizontal locking cabinet perfect for kitchens and reasonably priced.

However you do it, the key is to be aware of the potential and ability for small children to access your medications. There is a joke in the medical community that is based on truth: the elderly can't get into their childproof bottles, but their grandchildren can. So locks are the best idea.

Vitamins are a problem for three reasons:

1. We tend not to lock them up.

2. They are often made like candy for children to take without complaint. Although their vitamins may be in the form of gummy bears, don't make a big deal of them. Don't show your children the bottle with cartoon characters. Dispense them one at a time and only one a day. Never use them as a reward. Never accede to the pleas for a second. Finally, keep these in your locked cabinet. Don't assume that high on the kitchen shelf will work. One day when you least expect it, your toddler will climb onto the kitchen shelf and stand up. Remember: these are more apt to be a temptation than the plain-looking pills you take.

3. Vitamins sometimes contain iron, which can be toxic in the doses available in an average vitamin bottle. My advice is to buy children's vitamins without iron. Unless there is a real medical reason to do so (such as iron-deficiency anemia), buy adult vitamins without iron. Nothing else in the multivitamin carries the level of toxicity that iron does.

STOCKPILING OVER-THE-COUNTER MEDICINES

In the same way that you may be short of prescription medications, OTC (over-the-counter) medications may also become supply limited. The FDA wants to exert more and more control over nonprescription medications and vitamins and other nutriceuticals. And predictably, everything government touches becomes more expensive and harder to get. Do you get a sudden cold and become miserable at night due to a plugged nose? Or do you have trouble getting to sleep and take melatonin at bedtime? Think of all your routine supplements and add the OTC meds you routinely use; then add the ones I recommend for emergency self-care listed here and in appendix B.

TOP 10 OTC MEDICATIONS TO STORE

1. Aleve

2. Benadryl (diphenhydramine)

3. Cetirizine HCL (generic antihistamine)

4. Hydrocortisone cream

5. Afrin nasal spray

6. Omeprazole (antacid)

7. Miconazole nitrate 2% antifungal cream

8. Senokot S (for constipation)

9. Antibiotic ointment

10. Mylanta (immediate-relief antacid)

Supplements are individual. In appendix B, I summarize the ones that I believe everyone should take. But you should make your own personal list and keep them stocked up three to six months in advance.

Think of the routine afflictions that make you run to the drugstore. I use Afrin and antihistamines for my runny or stuffy nose on occasion. Antacids? A topical anti-itch cream? Headache meds? Sore throat lozenges? Go through your family and make a list of each member's needs—even if not common. I don't get colds very often, but three days of no sleep because of a clogged nose is no fun. And it usually happens at the most inopportune time. You want to develop a relationship with a freethinking non-government-dependent physician *before* the system collapses.

16

STOCKPILING AND DISTRIBUTING SUPPLIES

I once heard economist and investor Mark Faber, in referring to purchasing and holding physical gold, say that you should be like a dog and bury a bone in every backyard because you never know where you may end up. Now, he was referring to storing gold in different countries, but the principle is important for anything you might need in an emergency. Where will you be when you need the emergency item? If you have more than one house—say, a vacation cabin—it is important to have critical medical supplies anyplace you might end up during an emergency. Maybe the major supply cache is at home, but at least part of it should be in your vacation cabin or your "bolt hole." I keep a small house as a peripheral office eighty-two miles from my residence, and I am distributing some survival medical supplies there as well as the basics of food, clothing, and so on. And just as there are many types of survival guides, you should consider many types of supplies for different types of emergency. Classic "prepping" considers three levels of emergency: the seventy-two-hour evacuation, the six-week problem, and the long-haul survival scenario. Regarding medical supplies, I really envision only two types of supply kits. There is the really emergent small kit for the quick evacuation. And beyond that, medical organization should be by function, not time.

You will need to create (1) a small pack to get you by in a dire-straits, leave-in-minutes emergency; and (2) multiple problem–based supply units that are as complex as your level of medical knowledge and expertise.

THE TRUE EMERGENCY PANIC KIT

What would you grab to flee Hurricane Katrina, Mount St. Helens, or perhaps a forest fire, where you have less than thirty minutes to leave? This is when you grab your seventy-two-hour packs, your important documents, and your valuables if possible. And now let's add an emergency medical kit.

You can buy seventy-two-hour kits with basic first-aid supplies: Band-Aids, ACE bandages, salve, and so forth. But these won't come with your personal medicines, nor will they anticipate your particular needs if you have them—think diabetes. These standard seventy-two-hour kits (with food, water, candles, and such) are for surviving the first seventy-two hours. (See appendix B for representative contents of a seventy-two-hour kit.) It is assumed that there will be everyday supplies available after that. While it is true that nonmedical supplies, such as food and water, are pretty universal, medical care is not. So a seventy-two-hour emergency medical kit needs at least two weeks of medication in addition to basic first-aid items. One pack may work for a healthy family. But if people have medical care needs, everyone may need to evacuate with a seventy-two-hour pack *and* a medical pack. And remember that others you encounter along the way may need help. So this pack is not just for you; it is also to lend aid to those around you to some degree. The ability to help others is both good in itself and may provide a bartering tool if needed.

SHORT-TERM EMERGENCY PACKS

- ❏ Prescription medicines (in daily-dose ziplock snack bags—enough for at least two to three weeks)

- ❏ Chewable vitamin C

- ❏ Vitamin D_3

- ❏ Iodine supplement

- ❏ Melatonin 3 mg sublingual

- ❏ Antibiotic ointment

- ❏ Band-Aids

- ❏ Two or three (4-inch) ACE wraps

- ❏ A dozen 4 x 4-inch gauze bandages

- ❏ Cetirizine

- ❏ Hydrocortisone cream

- ❏ Q-tips (in a baggie)

- ❏ Aleve

- ❏ Afrin (nasal spray)

- ❏ N95 masks

- ❏ Cipro 500 or 750 mg tablets

- ❏ Clindamycin 300 mg tablets

- ❏ SAM Splint

- ❏ Sling

- ❏ Water purification tablets

- ❏ Special Ops manual

THE AMAL—LARGER SUPPLY BOXES

Any former US Navy medical personnel reading this will find humor in calling these supply boxes AMALs. AMALs—authorized medical allowance lists—were meant to be functional units. You had these big-boxed AMALs for general surgery, for medical clinics, and so on. But they tended to be packed wrong. To get an ear syringe, you would have to unpack pounds of gauze sponges. Or you might have to wade through pounds of ACE wraps to get a few Band-Aids. The Navy may have it figured out now, but that's the way it was when I was in the service. In our home medical preparation, we're going to do better by doing smaller. The bigger the package, the harder to get to what you need. But in the general concept, the idea of an AMAL makes some sense. Package items together by their function. In this case, if you want a good, orderly medical supply, I recommend using smaller, functional containers.

IMPORTANT AMALS TO HAVE ON HAND

- ❏ Prescription drugs

- ❏ Ointments/skin products

- ❏ Wound care items

- ❏ Splints

- ❏ Disinfectants and water purification tablets

- ❏ Information and testing equipment (nuclear/biologic/ chemical exposure items)

- ❏ Pet care items (optional)

- ❏ Respiratory care items (optional)

Do not use open bins. I made that mistake early on. These boxes should be stackable with secure lids, moisture proof, lightweight, and preferably clear so they are easy to search. Each should be clearly labeled and contain a list of items in the box to facilitate routine restocking. Rubbermaid makes a high-quality, good-sized box with a locking lid. But there are others on the market, and the Internet offers many options.

The items contained in the boxes should also reflect your level of medical expertise. (See appendix B for itemized contents of AMALs.) As a surgeon, I have two wound care AMALs: one for nonsurgical wound care—Band Aids, Neosporin, topical disinfectant, dressings and ACE wraps, tape—and a surgical add-on pack with suture, suturing kits, sterile drapes, and gloves. You need to keep your reference books handy, and the easiest thing is to put them in a box with your thermometer, blood pressure cuff, and stethoscope, if you have them. Remember that most new thermometers are battery powered and may go dead in your box or when you need them. I am hoarding my father's old mercury thermometers. In the absence of those, get the kind that do not require batteries. In other words, use the kind with alcohol or some other less accurate fluid the EPA will now allow us to use. (We can't get mercury thermometers, which are the best, but they force us to use mercury vapor bulbs, which require nine pages in the *Federal Register* outlining how to legally dispose of the toxic suckers.)

NUCLEAR EXPOSURE: MONITORING AND MEDICINE

It may sound paranoid, but these days I feel justified in some paranoia. As a medical provider living within twenty miles of a nuclear power plant, I bought a used, recalibrated FEMA Geiger counter—one of those yellow ones that were kept for possible nuclear attack. Ironically, in an age when we know nuclear plants can be compromised, FEMA got rid of the best testing devices. Many problems in a nuclear meltdown or bombing are caused by ignorance. As a medical provider,

I want to understand which areas are contaminated and which are safe. Unnecessary evacuation of one's home can be avoided, and mass evacuation can be avoided (or recommended in time) with the right knowledge. For radiation information I recommend the website Ki4U. com. They sell the easiest and cheapest tester—the RadSticker, which fits into your wallet. And they sell potassium iodide and other testing devices. Or you can also buy radiation stickers in small quantities at http://www.ush2.com/potassium_iodide_radiation_tools.htm. I keep all my radiation supplies in my "Information and Testing" AMAL (see appendix B).

POTASSIUM IODIDE (KI)

This is not a daily iodine supplement but a larger dose of iodine to prevent thyroid cancer when exposed to radiation, as happened to people near Fukushima and Chernobyl. Taken before the exposure, it is highly effective, and it is still 90 percent effective within two hours of exposure. Although the effectiveness degrades with time, because there is a risk of some ongoing exposure, I would take a single dose even a day or so after exposure. Generally take one dose as soon as a significant risk is known, and in prolonged exposure a daily dose for three days may be warranted—except in neonates and breast-feeding women. Keep in mind that adults over forty have less chance of thyroid cancer than younger people and a greater chance of allergy to KI. In the event of a radiation emergency, hopefully you will have some official source of information, but generally the government is too slow, in denial, and more worried about damage control for itself than damage control for you. Here are the dosing guidelines—understand that early action is best.

	PREDICTED THYROID EXPOSURE (cGy)	KI DOSE (MG)	NUMBER OR FRACTION OF 130 MG TABLETS	NUMBER OR FRACTION OF 65 MG TABLETS	MILLILITERS (ML) OF ORAL SOLUTION, 65 MG/ML
ADULTS OVER 40 YEARS	≥ 500**	130	1	2	2 ML
ADULTS OVER 18 THROUGH 40 YEARS	≥ 10**	130	1	2	2 ML
PREGNANT OR LACTATING WOMEN	≥ 5	130	1	2	2 ML
ADOLESCENTS, 12 THROUGH 18 YEARS*	≥ 5	65	½	1	1 ML
CHILDREN OVER 3 YEARS THROUGH 12 YEARS	≥ 5	65	½	1	1 ML
CHILDREN 1 MONTH THROUGH 3 YEARS	≥ 5	32	¼	½	0.5 ML
INFANTS BIRTH THROUGH 1 MONTH	≥ 5	16		¼	0.25 ML

*Adolescents approaching adult size (≥70 kg) should receive the full adult dose (130 mg).

**FDA understands that a KI administration program that sets different projected thyroid radioactive dose thresholds (committed dose equivalent (CDE)) for treatment of different population groups may be logistically impractical to implement during a radiological emergency.

SOURCE: Radiation Emergency Medical Management, DHS, http://www.remm.nlm.gov/potassiumiodide.htm

Finally, let me take this opportunity to criticize the current thinking on nuclear exposure. Although the information just given is most likely to be used in the event of a nuclear power plant accident, it is dangerous to ignore the possibility of a nuclear conflict between nation-states or a nuclear weapon being detonated by a nonstate actor, such as the current crop of terrorists. Although comedians and various talking heads make fun of the old nuclear drills done in the 1960s, the principles taught back then make sense and will save lives. (Many people think, mistakenly, that the chance of surviving is so low there is no reason to worry about learning such precautions.) In short, if you see a flash, drop under a desk or other object to avoid being struck by flying glass. Stay there for two minutes. Remember the 7:10 rule. Radiation loses 90 percent of its radioactivity in the first seven hours and 90 percent for every sevenfold interval of time, or 90 percent in seven hours, 99 percent in forty-nine hours, and 99.9 percent in fourteen days. Fallout looks like ash grit or sand. Place a white paper outside to check for it. No fallout, no radiation. Further information on radiation and other disaster medical preparedness can be found on the Doctors for Disaster Preparedness website, at http://www.ddponline.org. A handbook of emergency care in disaster scenarios can also be obtained from their site at http://www.ddponline.org/handbookforsurvival.pdf.

BIOLOGIC PRECAUTIONS

Unfortunately, although we may have reduced death from many childhood diseases, the world is an increasingly dangerous place. We may not be dying of malaria in the United States, but we are facing new threats from biologic agents of war and from the diseases being reintroduced by the hordes of illegal immigrants currently coming up from Central America. For these issues you need to be prepared for medical isolation if necessary.

BIOTERRORISM

After 9/11, I decided to educate myself about bioterrorism because my county health department spent $250,000 on a decontamination unit. My question was, what are they expecting to decontaminate? After enough research that I became a speaker on this topic, most recently giving a presentation to Doctors for Disaster Preparedness,

I still don't know what they planned on decontaminating. But I did learn there are some real issues out there, and we are sticking our collective national head in the sand.

The Obama administration, which claims to be the smartest group of political geniuses ever to grace the halls of American power, just got an F—for "Fail"—from Homeland Security for their inability to defend us against chemical or biologic attack. I, for one, was not surprised. For years I attempted to rouse then governor of Arizona Janet Napolitano to the dangers of biologic attack, and received no response. Failing at algebra is one thing, but the consequences of this failing grade could be the destruction of America and any other nation with its head in the sand on this issue. There are a handful of biologic agents that can be used as effective weapons. In most cases, either there is a treatment (such as with anthrax) or the disease is unlikely to spread (as with the botulinum toxin) or it is debilitating in the short term but not terribly deadly (in the case of salmonella). If, however, you want to pick a biologic agent that is very deadly, very communicable, and for which no treatment exists, you want smallpox.

SMALLPOX

The United States stopped routine smallpox vaccinations in 1972, the last known natural case occurring in 1967. Smallpox is an unbelievably deadly disease. It is the most contagious disease known to mankind—spreading literally like smoke. In the last known outbreak in Europe, a man early in the throes of smallpox, against doctor's advice, opened his hospital window. In the cold German night, his exhalations went out the window, up the hospital wall, into an open window on another wing, and killed several nurses. That's contagious.

Smallpox is a virus for which there is no known treatment, and in some outbreaks the death rate for those infected was over 60 percent. Modern medicine brought the contagion under control by a process of "ring vaccination." The Centers for Disease Control

(CDC), the World Health Organization (WHO), and other agencies prepositioned vaccine at hot spots all over the world. They had trained teams of medical personnel ready to go at a moment's notice to fly to any area suffering an outbreak and begin vaccinating people in a ring around the incident case until the outbreak stopped.

While it is true that smallpox has been eradicated in the wild, it is not gone. As smallpox came under some control, samples from the disease were given to the CDC in Atlanta and to Biopreparat/Vector in the Soviet Union. Just as Oppenheimer thought it would be a more stable world if both sides had nuclear bombs, the WHO thought it was only fair that both the democratic United States and the totalitarian Soviets should have samples of the world's deadliest disease.

We know for a fact that when Nixon signed the treaty with the Soviets in the early 1970s to halt all offensive bioweapons research and deployment, the Russians went right home and created the largest bioweapons program known to mankind. According to Ken Alibek (his Americanized name), himself a defector and the number-two man at Vector State Research Center of Virology and Biotechnology, the Soviet Union had vats filled with more than twenty tons of India-11 smallpox that had been prepared for delivery in warheads. Our intelligence services had witnessed testing of ICBM reentry vehicles with nose-cone cooling, something needed only for bioagents. And we know that at the fall of the Soviet empire, the bioweaponeers disappeared, along with their agents—presumably to the highest bidder.

So here is the scenario in a nutshell. Smallpox virus survives in freezers all over the world—not just in friendly hands. We found incubation vats in Iraq labeled "smallpox," and we captured Saddam's bioweaponeer, a woman fondly referred to as Dr. Germ. The virus that was manufactured by the Soviets was about 60 percent lethal, and the amount to start a worldwide contagion may be stored in a single chicken egg. Before, disease containment was possible because (1) much of the developed world was vaccinated, (2) teams trained to handle outbreaks were standing by for ready deployment worldwide, (3) vaccine was stashed in accessible depots all over the world, (4) populations were less mobile, and (5) people knew not to go to hospitals during smallpox outbreaks but to allow a system of quarantine. But today, none of these things is true; and additionally, since the 1970s, we have the scientific wherewithal to genetically modify (weaponize) the virus.

I served in the military and have had a number of smallpox vaccinations. Unfortunately, these probably last only fifteen years. As a trauma surgeon and emergency responder, I tried to be voluntarily vaccinated but was turned down. At that time, Janet Reno was governor of Arizona, and she was worried that voluntary vaccination of hospital personnel might result in workman's compensation claims. How do you spell shortsighted? Since 9/11, I have written to two governors and numerous health agencies, expressing my fear about the deadliest terrorist weapon—biologic agents, particularly smallpox. My request was a simple one—let the first responders be voluntarily inoculated against smallpox. At present only a handful of people in county health departments are vaccinated.

BIOWEAPON	DEADLY?	COMMUNICABLE?	CURE?
EBOLA	YES	ONLY WITH DIRECT CONTACT	NO
ANTHRAX	YES	NOT USUALLY	YES (CIPRO / DOXYCYCLINE)
BOTULINUM TOXIN	YES	NO	NO
TULAREMIA	YES	NO	YES (CIPRO / DOXYCYCLINE)
PLAGUE	YES	NO	YES (PENICILLIN)
SMALLPOX*	YES*	YES*	NO*

*Only smallpox is deadly, communicable, and without cure.

So, in the case of a bioweapon being released, to be prepared, first you need to be knowledgeable because the news will not tell you the whole or even the true story should this occur. Don't panic for outbreaks of influenza, anthrax, ebola, or pretty much any other bioterrorist weapon—unless you hear the word *smallpox*. If there is even one case of smallpox reported anywhere in the world, it is cause for action. The only action you can take is to isolate yourself. I have told my family that should smallpox break out anywhere in the world, within days of the report it will be global. Do not get on any public transportation. It is time to get to a freestanding domicile, preferably a rural one, that has enough supplies to last several months. I won't repeat classic survivalist instruction here, but suffice it to say that this is the one situation in which secure isolation is the safest solution. You cannot allow any potentially contaminated people near you. I hope that public health will be able to distribute the vaccine and that there will be house-to-house vaccination or some other sort of community vaccination program. Keep in mind that vaccination pre-exposure is essentially 100 percent effective in preventing the disease. Vaccination after exposure mitigates death but does not completely diminish the chance of contracting this disfiguring disease. In your stored medications I have recommended both cipro and doxicycline as treatment. Most masks will not screen out smallpox, but they may help with other communicable diseases such as TB (see below). For this purpose you should have a box of N95 masks in appropriate sizes, and keep them at home, in your car, and in your emergency kits.

Illegal immigrants now swarming the southern border from El Salvador, Honduras, and Guatemala are bringing with them a panoply of diseases that, up until now, have been rare in the United States or had been eradicated. Although legal immigration required testing for a number of communicable diseases, illegals gain entry without any such precaution. If unchecked, this latest assault on our border integrity will become not only a crime problem but a public health disaster.

DISEASES OF ILLEGAL IMMIGRATION

1. Multidrug-resistant TB

2. Chagas disease

3. Leprosy

4. Measles

5. Influenza

6. Malaria

7. Dengue fever

8. Hepatitis A, B, C, E

9. Lice, scabies, and other parasites

Tuberculosis (TB) was once very common but had been controlled in the United States through testing and public health measures. Prior to anti-TB meds, 2 percent of medical students died during training due to patient exposure to the disease. Today about two million people worldwide die yearly from TB, and now we are facing an influx of the very worst strain of the disease brought in through illegal immigration. Multiple-drug-resistant TB requires very expensive medications to be given—often through IV—sometimes for years. Even so, it carries a 50 percent chance of premature death and costs from $250,000 to $1.2 million to treat one patient. Currently, a good number of the immigrants reaching and crossing the border are sick with one or more of these diseases. They are coughing up blood, and they are malnourished and infested with body lice and parasites. The border patrol agents trying to control the problem are being infected.[1] At the time of this writing, the nationwide impact of this disaster has yet to play out, so clear recommendations are difficult. In general, optimize your vitamin

D levels and your general health to be resistant to disease as much as possible. Keep N95 masks—which were designed specifically to filter out TB particles—handy for unexpected situations. Keep cipro and doxycycline in your medical stores, along with treatment for lice (Quell). If you are going to be hospitalized, especially if this is elective and you have the luxury of rescheduling, ask about cases of TB and whether or not such cases are in the hospital. The sad fact is, in the old days we had sanatoriums where we isolated TB victims and applied "open-air treatment." These are all closed. Today, modern non-research hospitals rarely have true isolation rooms. They can put the TB patient into a single-bed room, but the air that circulates through the room also circulates around into other patients' rooms. So having your gall bladder surgery could get you exposed to a bad disease—if this crisis spreads.

There is nothing good to say about the potential threats facing us medically in an increasingly unstable modern world. Ironically, the government is regulating us to the point that we are losing our scientific and medical edge. But the Obama administration is failing in its one constitutionally mandated function of protecting the American people against invasion. And the medical result of that failure is yet to be fully manifest.

EBOLA

Ebola (named after the Ebola River in Zaire) is a very fatal disease of African origin. It is a long fibrous-appearing virus that is spread only by direct contact. Known as "hemorrhagic fever" because those affected bleed from every orifice, the disease is manifest within ten days of exposure, often much earlier. Depending on population and access to care, disease fatality ranges from 20 to 90 percent, and there is no treatment except supportive care. However, this disease is easily controllable by quarantine since it is not airborne. Before the paving of the Kinshasa highway, which increased access to remote villages, people from endemic areas of deepest sub-Saharan Africa might have been wiped out, but it would not have spread. Now an infected person can drive or be driven to unaffected areas more easily and spread the disease. The disease manifests generally within 72 hours from exposure. If a small outbreak in America does occur, simply stay away from people outside your immediate family until the outbreak is controlled. The degree of isolation and/or need for isolation is related to the degree of outbreak. Duct taping windows, Hazmat suits, gas masks, and the like are unnecessary because this virus is not airborne.

ROTATION OF SUPPLIES

Stockpiling supplies means keeping things fresh and rotating items. The only things you really need to worry about in this regard are the medications. Elastic bandages and sticky bandages, such as Band-Aids, will degrade over the years, but if kept at room temperature in a closet or basement, these items will last decades. As noted previously, shelf life of most medications is also over five years.

As you add medications to your stockpile, put a label on the outside of your stored medicine bin that lists the contents by name and the date of expiration. Use small return address labels, one per medicine; and as you replace drugs, simply make a new sticker and put it over the old. Don't be tempted to write with magic marker directly on the bin. I did that, and as things changed, the bin got too scratched out and written over. (In fact, in my experience, writing directly on storage bins doesn't even work with simple things like Christmas decorations.)

Some of the medications you store you hope you never use. But then there are also stores of medications you do use. As noted earlier, due to the uncertainty of the supply in the future, it is prudent to keep on hand three to six months' worth of the meds you use regularly. Store these medications where they are easily accessible—either in a separate bin or on top of all the ones you don't plan on using often. Every time you refill your prescription, add the new meds to the box, and use the oldest in the box for that month. And of course, medications that need to stay cool should be stored in the refrigerator. If in doubt, ask your pharmacist.

EpiPens, because they may be lifesaving, need to be scattered around your life—purse, desk drawer at work, kitchen cabinet, and so on. If you are at high risk of anaphylactic airway constriction, it doesn't help to have your EpiPen buried deep in a storage box. Because they really do expire shortly after the given expiration date, make sure to use them or replace them by the date indicated. Any in a storage box must be kept handy and rotated on time!

17

REAL EMERGENCIES THAT CAN'T WAIT

I t is critical to determine when you can temporize a medical problem with a "wait and see" attitude, possibly avoiding an unnecessary trip to the doctor, or when you have to go *now*. In the following chapters we will explore home care for a variety of things in depth. But some things just have to receive some level of professional help. These are some of the things you cannot afford to self-treat beyond initial emergency care:

- Airway obstruction (significant difficulty breathing)

- Compromised circulation

- Progressive numbness or weakness (possible stroke)

- Open fractures (bone through skin)

- Dislocation (that can't be reduced)

- Penetrating wound to a joint

- Chest pain (possible heart attack)

- Loss of consciousness or changed mental status

- Poisoning

- Venomous human and animal bites

- Fever with other symptoms

- Spontaneous bleeding

- Inability to urinate or defecate (have bowel movement)

- Abdominal pain

AIRWAY OBSTRUCTION

An airway obstruction should always be taken seriously. There are two types of "obstruction": (1) inhalation of an object and (2) intrinsic airway collapse or constriction. Sometimes the source is obvious: your kid swallows a quarter and it lodges in the trachea, and he can barely breathe. Sometimes it is not: your kid complains of shortness of breath but seems to be moving his chest and moving air. An airway problem is so critical that you should err on the side of caution.

When we say "airway obstruction," we include in our thinking asthma and other forms of constriction that are not caused by a foreign body such as a quarter. Asthma "obstructs" the airway by squeezing closed the tubes in the lungs that allow air to pass. If asthma runs in the family and your child complains she can't breathe and her airways are clear, an asthma inhaler may provide temporary relief. If you don't have an inhaler, you can try taking a hot shower. The steam relaxes the airways. Fast-acting allergy medicine like Benadryl or Claritin might help, as many asthma attacks are triggered by allergies. Caffeine is another trick to opening constricted airways. A couple of cups of coffee or cans of soda might be enough to find relief. But if symptoms persist or continue to worsen, you need to seek medical attention immediately.

If asthma is not the culprit and you are not sure what is happening, look around the collarbone near the neck. Any skin sinking in toward the lung with attempts at breathing is called "retraction" and is a sign of respiratory distress. Put your ear to the chest. Do you hear air moving? Are there wheezes? Is there a hornlike sound as air squeaks around the quarter or Lego or other inhaled object?

If you know there is a physical obstruction to the airway, then attempt to clear it out. The classic obstruction is food. A person is eating in the restaurant and starts to choke. He cannot talk and makes the sign for choking (at least in theory). In spite of what you may have heard, DO NOT HIT HIM ON THE BACK. Banging on the back only serves to lodge the food or other obstruction even more deeply. There are total obstructions where the patient cannot speak and cannot breathe, and partial obstructions where he cannot talk but can still cough or breathe around the obstruction. If possible, in a partial airway obstruction, invert the person and let this clear the obstruction. When the head is down, there is a natural tendency for the airway to relax and allow the food or toy to work itself out. (This is something a person can try if alone and choking.) This is a great move for a choking child who can be held upside down.

The classic maneuver is the abdominal squeeze—two quick thrusts upward at the base of the sternum that forces the air to propel the obstruction out. That can be done with the patient upright or on the floor if unconscious. Taking a first aid/CPR course is a good idea to really learn this technique (and the technique for CPR).

In sum, when in doubt about a person who is having trouble breathing, seek help early. This is not

NONEMERGENCIES THAT NEED ATTENTION:

- Sprains
- Migraines
- Stomachaches
- Minor fever
- Earaches
- Minor wounds (not requiring stitches)
- Sore throats
- Tick bites
- Minor eye injury
- Insomnia
- Hypertension
- Diarrhea

a problem where you "wait and see." Better to arrive at an ER and not need to be seen, than to wait too long and turn a small problem into a catastrophe. As a personal example, years ago, I took my two-year-old to the ER in the middle of the night because of an asthma-like attack. He was suddenly audibly wheezing and had retractions of the chest as described earlier. Until this time no one in the family needed any asthma treatment, so I had no medications and could do nothing at home. I put him in the car and raced off to the ER. But after the ten minutes it took to get to the ER, probably thanks to the cool air and a little bit of excitement-induced adrenaline, he was almost normal. We waited and waited to be seen by the ER doctor, and during this time my young son toddled out into the hall and said loudly, "If no one is coming, I'm going home!" As a doctor who is usually on the other end of such complaints, I had to laugh. And now we have experience (and medicine) for just such an emergency.

COMPROMISED CIRCULATION

There are many older people who have a long history of diminished circulation characterized by cool feet, hairless toes, and chronic skin darkening. They may occasionally have a bluish toe, which should be under the care of a vascular surgeon. Usually this situation is already known and is not an emergency. Similarly, one may have a cold, pale, or bluish finger or toe or foot from cold exposure. This can usually be treated by warming the extremity and is usually not a critical emergency.

An emergency is a sudden pale, cold, pulseless extremity without clear cause. This is often due to trauma. Any injury with swelling that seems to be cutting off circulation is critical. It is important in this situation to restore the general alignment of the extremity and splint the limb. Occasionally, a clot will form in an artery and cause a limb to lose circulation. In these settings, while you are getting to definitive medical care, icing the extremity will increase the time the limb can survive without blood circulation. A limb can last one and a half hours without circulation. After that, ice extends the survival time. If you need several hours to reach higher-level care, icing will improve the chance of limb salvage.

Another true emergency is a suddenly swollen leg—and I mean obviously swollen and usually painful, *without known cause*. A sprained ankle or significant bang to the shin can give you swelling but is not a flat-out emergency. Swelling of a leg without clear cause may be due to DVT—deep venous thrombosis—a blood clot in the deep veins of the legs. This is serious both for the leg and for the fact that the clot may break apart and move into the lung. A clot in the lung can cause severe oxygen deprivation or heart failure and thereby cause death. Leg clots are more apt to happen to people recently immobilized in a cast or other constricting device, or to people who are bedridden, who smoke, or who have a history of blood clots in their legs or lungs. There is no home remedy for this problem, and you need to seek help. Taking a baby aspirin is a good idea while arranging transport. Keep the leg elevated, and don't walk around.

RISK FACTORS FOR BLOOD CLOTS

- Cancer or other chronic illness
- Cast, brace, or other immobilization
- Long-distance plane travel
- History of clotting problem
- Prolonged bed rest
- Smoking

PROGRESSIVE NUMBNESS OR WEAKNESS (POSSIBLE STROKE)

A stroke or cerebrovascular accident (CVA) is due to altered blood to the brain. This can present with slurred speech, sudden altered mental status, or weakness or numbness of the extremities or face, usually on one side of the body. Use the F.A.S.T. (Face, Arms, Speech, Time) test to see if someone is having a stroke. Ask her to smile, to raise her hands above her head, to speak, and to stick out her tongue. Look for drooping eye or mouth, inability to raise one hand, inability to speak, or deviation of the tongue to one side. Symptoms of a ministroke include minor motor dysfunction or weakness on one side of the body, diminished vision and/or light sensitivity in one eye, and a severe headache. Sometimes you are having a transient ischemic attack, or TIA, and these resolve over twenty-four hours. But you cannot know this ahead of time. If you are experiencing symptoms of a stroke or someone else notices your slurred speech or lopsided face, there are three things you *must not do*:

1. Do not delay in getting help at a hospital.

2. Do not take an aspirin (some strokes may be from bleeding, and this will worsen it).

3. Do not drive yourself.

Progressive neurologic deficit without evidence of stroke—in other words, loss of nerve function, such as weakness, confusion, or decreased sensation that occurs over hours—is rare, but it can happen in spinal cord disease or herniated disks. You should seek emergent care if the person experiences progressive weakness or numbness over hours or days. For example, if a person has back pain radiating into a leg, then has weakness of the foot, and later that day weakness of the leg, that is "progressive deficit," and the patient needs transport to a hospital. Any numbness around the rectum or vagina or loss of control of bowel or bladder (meaning leaking stool and urine) that comes on over hours or days also requires emergent evaluation.

OPEN FRACTURES

Later in the book you will learn home care for routine fractures. But some fractures cannot wait and must be cared for in an emergency department. An open, or compound, fracture is one in which the bone comes through the skin—however slightly. If not treated with a surgical procedure to open and wash out the wound and remove contaminated bone within six hours, the rate of deep bone infection rises significantly. Seek professional orthopaedic help.

If you cannot get to help, the next best thing is to flush the wound/bone with several quarts of clean or sterile water with a tiny bit of pure soap or antibacterial soap added. Then make sure the limb has good blood flow—if necessary, by pulling it straighter. Next, cover the wound with a sterile dressing with antibiotic ointment underneath and/or Betadine in the dressing. Apply a splint (see chapter 22). If you have cipro in your medicine cabinet, this is the time to take 750 milligrams while awaiting definitive care. Children are more difficult to dose. Cipro is not recommended for children. For children, I would use clindamycin as soon as possible when delay in definitive care is established. Clindamycin dosage is 40 mg/kg/day in three to four divided doses (see sidebar). Keep in mind these recommendations are not the standard medical approved therapy. This is the fallback plan when the correct hospital-based physician care is not available.

CLINDAMYCIN DOSAGE CHART FOR CHILDREN

When definitive care is not available and you need to treat an open fracture in a child, consider treating with clindamycin for no more than three days while awaiting hospital care.

CHILD'S WEIGHT	DOSE	FREQUENCY
20 POUNDS	150 MG CAPSULE	EVERY 8 HOURS
30 POUNDS	150 MG CAPSULE	EVERY 6 HOURS
40 POUNDS OR MORE	300 MG	EVERY 8 HOURS

DISLOCATIONS

Anyone who has played contact sports has probably had or seen a dislocation—usually a finger or a shoulder. It is often possible to reduce dislocations immediately after they happen while the tissues are still a little numb from the trauma. In general the principle is to reproduce the deformity, then pull straight. For example, if a finger is dislocated and the end of the finger is sticking up at the first joint, you (or usually someone else) pull the finger up more and keeping tension on the finger, allow it to relocate into a straight alignment. In other words, first pull in line with the dislocated part.

Many people have dislocated shoulders, and these are a little more complicated. The easiest thing to do is to lie facedown on a table or high bed, letting your arm hang over the side. Put a rolled-up towel or firm pad under the chest just next to the shoulder, but not under the shoulder. Hold or tape a weight—ten to fifteen pounds—to your hand. Relax and let gravity put the shoulder back into place. Alternatively, this technique can be used with your friend (hopefully he will still be your friend after this experience) doing the pulling instead of using a weight. If you have any Valium (10- to 15-milligram tablet for an adult), take it ten minutes before this procedure to aid in relaxation.

The key to reduction of a shoulder is not brute force but relaxation of the person injured. When I was a first-year orthopaedic resident on trauma call, I walked into the "cast room" and witnessed five big orthopaedic guys—four residents and the chief of the department—pulling on the arm and applying countertraction to the chest of an old man with a shoulder dislocation. More than six hundred pounds of combined muscle could not reduce the shoulder. But the female resident (me) then took the patient to the OR where, under general anesthesia, it took literally three fingers to reduce the shoulder dislocation because the patient was relaxed. I always remember the incident, both for the dramatically easy reduction and because the minute the shoulder dropped into place, the whole floor started waving and moving in a thirty-second earthquake.

If the dislocation is reduced, great! Now you can follow up as needed in the daylight hours with an orthopaedic surgeon. If you can't reduce it, or are unsure—head for emergency help.

PENETRATING WOUND TO A JOINT

Unless you are a gangbanger and at risk for gunshot wounds, any joint penetrations you get will probably be from the knife slipping or your friendly cat. Any puncture wound to a joint from any cause has contaminated the joint with bacteria, and you cannot treat that at home. Seek help.

CHEST PAIN (POSSIBLE HEART ATTACK)

It is easier to say what is usually not a heart attack, but again, one can be fooled. Generally, if you are in a low-risk group—under fifty, a nonsmoker, without significant medical problems, and do not have classic symptoms—you are unlikely to be having a heart attack. If you can push on your chest wall and reproduce the pain, it is probably not a heart attack. If it goes away with a little antacid, it is probably not a heart attack. However, heart attacks are difficult even for seasoned emergency room doctors to sort out, so when in doubt, don't hesitate to get help.

The classic symptoms of a heart attack include deep chest pressure or pain (often characterized as an elephant standing on one's chest), sweating, radiation of achy pain to the jaw or arm, shortness of breath, light-headedness, nausea, or vomiting. Unfortunately all or none may be present. We miss many "silent" heart attacks that are totally asymptomatic and are picked up later on EKG. And many heart attacks have only one symptom or are atypical. One symptom I would never ignore is the feeling of doom or foreboding. Some people report a sense of death or doom and were found to have a subtle but life-threatening disorder. I took myself to the ER when I was twenty-two, worried about my heart. In retrospect, it was a lot of subconscious, uninformed fear from my father dying of heart disease two years earlier, combined with pain in the cartilage joints in my chest—costochondritis. However, you should always listen to your subconscious when it feels seriously threatened.

Nonsmokers under forty generally don't die from a heart attack. If they have a painful heart condition, it is usually a muscular or ligamentous or joint cartilage–type chest pain, which isn't a heart attack but which shouldn't be ignored either. I would be more worried about smokers over forty, anyone over fifty, and anyone with the classic symptoms.

If you do think it is your heart, call an ambulance or have someone prepare to drive you to an emergency room. Take a baby aspirin as soon as you can, as this can prevent clotting within the coronary (heart) arteries and has been shown to decrease damage and reduce the likelihood of death. But only take one baby aspirin. In this case more is not better.

Sadly, sometimes the first presentation of heart disease is sudden death. If someone collapses and is pulseless, institute CPR per the latest protocol. It should be noted that the protocols are written these days not for the optimal result but so that people will not fail to start CPR. In other words, it has become "CPR for Dummies and the Reluctant." You can review the following CPR illustrations. But in days past we did several things not mentioned here. When we witnessed a person collapsing, we first administered a "precordial thump"—a bang on the chest directly over the heart. In cases of a rhythm problem where the electrical starter of the heart malfunctions, this can restart the heart. It works; and if I drop over, please do that for me. *But* it was taken out of the protocol because people were thumping over and over rather than beginning the messier breathing, pushing CPR. So if you give a thump, ONLY DO IT ONCE; then move on. Similarly, CPR used to include mouth-to-mouth breathing for the patient, to provide better oxygenation. This was taken out because people were reluctant to put their mouths on strangers and so failed to start CPR. But trust me—I have firsthand experience here—it is much more effective to intersperse mouth-to-mouth breaths between chest compressions. The latest recommended ratio is two breaths per thirty chest compressions, and the chest compressions should be done at the rate of one hundred compressions per minute.

CPR GUIDE

1. Assess the situation for danger, and if safe, tell any onlookers to call 911 for help.

2. See if the patient is responsive. Shake gently and ask loudly if they are okay.

3. If you have been trained and know how to apply a defibrillator ask another bystander to get any nearby defibrillator.

4. Check for breathing. Don't do this for more than 10 to 15 seconds. Look for chest rise and/or feel for air movement.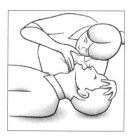

5. If the patient isn't breathing, begin chest compressions. Place the heel of your palm on the lower sternum (breastbone). Interlock your fingers of the other hand over the first one and push with both arms outstretched.

6. Begin chest compressions, depressing the chest two inches for a rate of 100 beats per minute. You can estimate this by pressing to the beat of the Bee Gees song "Staying Alive."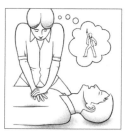

7. If possible have another bystander begin breathing at a rate of approximately two breaths per 20 compressions. You can do it yourself as well, but it is much easier with two people performing CPR. (Although they now teach a no-breathing technique, trust me, breathing is better for the victim when possible.)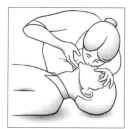

RECOGNIZE THE SIGNS

❑ Immense pressure on your chest

❑ Sweating

❑ Pain in the jaw or arm

❑ Shortness of breath

❑ Light-headedness

❑ Nausea

❑ Vomiting

PROTECT YOUR HEART THE "ANTI-AGING" WAY

❑ Don't smoke. If you smoke, quit as soon as possible.

❑ Eat only good natural fats: olive oil, coconut oil, animal fat, butter. Do not use man-made fats, such as Crisco, corn oil, or margarine.

❑ Take the essential supplements outlined in appendix B.

❑ Avoid gluten and generally eat low-carb.

❑ Get regular exercise, especially weight training.

❑ Keep your hormones at youthful levels through supplementation when indicated.

LOSS OF CONSCIOUSNESS OR CHANGED MENTAL STATUS

Anyone with an altered mental status for no apparent reason needs medical evaluation. While waiting to get to the hospital or awaiting transport, it is important to look for clues—change in skin color, shortness of breath, a new odor to the breath. There are whole books written about the diagnosis of altered mentation or coma, so you are not in the position of always sorting this out. But there are steps to take:

1. While waiting for transport, make sure to remove any constricting clothing.

2. If possible apply oxygen.

3. If the patient is awake and will not choke, drink clear water to rehydrate.

4. Since the brain blood flow may be compromised, it makes sense to keep the head only slightly above horizontal, so have the person reclining.

5. If the patient is a known diabetic, it is important to give him or her orange juice or something to raise the blood sugar.

6. Look for clues for accidental poisoning (see below).

7. Assemble the patient's medications for transport with her as well as her medical record (see appendix D for creating the personal medical record).

POISONING

In cases of poisoning or suspected poisoning, call the Poison Control Center at 1-800-222-1222. If the substance is caustic (see sidebar "Caustic Household Chemicals"), rinse the mouth with a little water or milk to remove any caustic chemical residue and seek medical help immediately. Caustic substances appear to burn the mouth and are associated with swelling, drooling, and painful swallowing. These are difficult to deal with, and *the only safe thing to do is to give clear water to dilute the substance.* All other recommendations here apply to NON-CAUSTIC poisons.

While waiting for the doctor, if the substance is not caustic (see sidebar "Common Nontoxic Substances") and very damaging to tissues, try to induce vomiting. (This is not very effective as time passes, and it does not get rid of all the stomach's contents.) This can be done by inserting fingers in the mouth and either pushing the tongue backward or touching the back of the throat. You can drink a warm mustard solution (see below). Any patient who is vomiting or trying to vomit should either be over a receptacle or on his side. DO NOT INDUCE VOMITING WHILE THE VICTIM IS ON HIS BACK BECAUSE HE MAY INHALE THE VOMIT.

Better than that home remedy is to have some activated charcoal at home (about a 15gm bottle) and give that as soon as possible. This may cause vomiting, but it is the best thing to inactivate many poisons. Even if charcoal is given, seek attention unless you can get definitive advice from a poison center. Do not use activated charcoal for caustic substances. Every passage of the substance through the mouth and esophagus increases contact time and possibly the chemical "burn."

> **MUSTARD DRINK**
> 1 tablespoon mustard
> 1 cup warm water
> Mix well with a spoon and drink rapidly to induce vomiting.

> **CAUSTIC HOUSEHOLD CHEMICALS**
> Ammonia
> Bleach
> Carpet shampoo
> Dishwasher detergent
> Drain cleaner
> Fingernail polish
> Kerosene
> Mold and mildew cleaners
> Oven cleaner
> Toilet bowl cleaner

VENOMOUS BITES

Most bites are harmless. Some become infected on a delayed basis. And some are accompanied by *envenomation*, or the injection of a toxic substance that causes death of the surrounding tissues or even patient death.

It is normal to have a red mark and swelling after an insect bite (think the standard mosquito bite). But if you have been bitten by a spider, scorpion, insect, or snake, such as a rattlesnake that is known to be venomous, or you start to experience any systemic

COMMON NONTOXIC SUBSTANCES

Bubble bath

Crayons

Chalk

Candles

Deodorant

Eye makeup

Household bleach

Laundry detergent

Lipstick

Lotion

Perfume

Play-Doh

Silly Putty

Soap

Toothpaste

Watercolors

symptoms after the bite, such as sweating, numbness, fevers or chills, shortness of breath, vomiting, facial swelling, tingling or numbness of the extremity, or progressive swelling near the bite, seek help because these bites need antivenom emergently. Call the poison center at 1-800-222-1222 and/or 911 to be directed to the nearest facility with antivenom. DO NOT APPLY ICE to envenomations from anything—snake or spider. Ice activates the venom and makes things worse. Keep the limb at heart level, and rush to the nearest antivenom facility. If possible, splint the extremity, being careful to allow for swelling. Remove all rings and any constricting bracelets. You can wash the area in soap and water, but do not try to "suck out the venom," as this puts the venom under your tongue, where it may be even better absorbed.

EMERGENCY CARE FOR VENOMOUS BITE WOUND

1. Call Poison Control at 1-800-222-1222 or 911 to find the closest facility with antivenom.

2. Arrange transportation; do not drive yourself.

3. Remove all rings and constricting bracelets or clothing.

4. DO NOT APPLY ICE.

5. Elevate the extremity slightly above the heart and rest it. Splint if possible.

6. Do not enlarge the wounds or suck out the venom.

Cats are notorious for puncturing small joints in the hand or the tendon sheaths with their little sharp, pointed teeth. This can result in deep hand infections. The problem may develop over twelve hours or several days. The same can be said for human "bites" because they often involve the knuckles (as in punching someone in the mouth) or become infected due to the strange bacteria that we harbor in our mouths. Any generalized redness or swelling after such a bite should be evaluated professionally. Any small, local redness and swelling can be observed and treated with frequent warm soaks (at least three times a day) and antibiotic cream or ointment. Bites from animals, such as dogs, ferrets, hamsters, or gerbils, are much less likely to cause joint penetration or deep infection because of the nature of their teeth and the germs in their mouths.

Finally, there is the issue of rabies. Rabies deaths in the United States are rare—fewer than ten a year. But forty thousand people are exposed and vaccinated. The vaccine is 100 percent effective at preventing the disease—even after exposure—but the disease is 100 percent fatal if contracted from a rabid animal. (Exposure to the disease is not the same as contracting the disease.) Rabies occurs quite often in populations of raccoons, foxes, skunks, coyotes, bobcats, woodchucks (groundhogs), beavers, and other large carnivores. Small mammals, such as squirrels, rats, mice, hamsters, guinea pigs, gerbils, chipmunks, rabbits, and hares are almost never found to be infected with rabies and have not been known to cause rabies among humans in the United States. Rabies is rarely seen in domestic cats and dogs, but these bites account for more rabies testing because fewer people are bitten by woodchucks.[1]

Any bite by a wild animal should be reported to the local health department or discussed with an emergency physician. Local health departments are given updates on rabies probability and protocols, and they can give the best advice. If that help is not available, it is critical to observe the vaccinated animal for ten days, an unvaccinated animal forty-five days. If there is no sign of rabies at that point, then no further treatment is needed.

Bats pose a different problem.[2] Of the approximately ten deaths a year from rabies, most are from exposure to a rabid bat. Any contact with a bat is of concern because the virus can be transmitted through superficial wounds or mucous membranes. If a bat is found in a house and if the possibility exists of unrecognized direct contact—for example, a sleeping baby in the room with the bat—it is best to capture the bat and call the local authorities. All wounds from bats must be considered rabid until proven otherwise. If the bat cannot be captured and there is any question of contact, the current recommendation is to vaccinate the potential victim. Symptoms of rabies generally occur two months after exposure, and vaccination even weeks after exposure prevents the disease. Should the medical care system collapse temporarily, you will have time to sort this out and possibly be able to locate rabies vaccine when needed.

Human bites are a problem because of the bad germs we carry in our mouths. If there is contamination of mouth germs to the wound or if the wound is ragged, deep, or puncturing or in the hand or tendons, you are best advised to seek help. If that is not available, cleanse the wound and leave it open—do not attempt to close a human bite. Cipro and clindamycin in combination may ward off infection. It is important never to lie to your treating physician about these wounds even though they frequently involve a fistfight where the knuckles hit the other combatant's tooth. Without knowing that fact, the doctor may undertreat the injury and a serious infection could ensue.

FEVER WITH OTHER SIGNS OR SYMPTOMS

Fever causes many unnecessary trips to emergency rooms. By itself, it is the body's adaptive response to infection. Fever is, in most cases, our friend. Much evidence suggests we should never use drugs to lower the fever because doing so prolongs the illness or increases the chance of death and disability. Years ago, studies were done in India using various antipyretics—temperature-lowering drugs—in children with tuberculosis (TB) or with polio. In cases of TB, those given diclofenac or aspirin to lower their temperature were found to have a higher death rate and a longer course of active disease before the body walled off the invading germs. In polio cases, similarly, paralysis and death were increased by chemically lowering the temperature. Because chemicals that lower temperature also alter the body's immune response, we cannot generalize these findings to lowering temperature mechanically. In other words, using grandma's method of lowering the temperature by tepid water baths and sponging, or putting on a moist T-shirt for evaporation, may not make things worse, but we do not know for sure. My approach is to tolerate most temperatures for as long as possible, and only when truly miserable do I sponge down or do the wet T-shirt trick.

So when do we go to the ER? If the fever is accompanied by other significant symptoms—such as severe headache, neck stiffness, change in mental status, unremitting nausea and vomiting, vision changes, seizures, generalized rash, severe abdominal pain or distention, or worse—go to the ER, calling 911 if needed.

If the fever is over 104 and persistent in spite of cooling, go to your physician or the local emergency room for evaluation. Even as a physician I believe in instinct. Instinct is really just your subconscious mind putting all the facts together, but not making you aware of the ongoing logic. There is a big difference between a child with a temperature of 104 who looks good, acts right, and whose temperature is easily brought down through sponge baths, and a child who appears very ill, is listless, and whose temperature does not respond to home remedies. The former I would feel comfortable watching at home. The latter I would take to the emergency room.

SPONTANEOUS BLEEDING
Many times when we are bleeding, we know what caused it. Sometimes, though, people can spontaneously start bleeding. Usually it is out of the nose. It is very common for kids to have nosebleeds,

maybe even several. But any bleeding that is unstoppable from the nose after a reasonable period of direct pressure should be taken in for professional packing and evaluation. An old-fashioned treatment for nosebleed, which has made a comeback, is packing with salt pork. For some reason cured pork packed into the nose stops bleeding even in people with bleeding disorders.

STOPPING A NOSEBLEED

1. Sit down and pinch your nose for at least 10 minutes (without peeking to see if the bleeding has stopped). Set your watch to confirm the time.

2. Keep the head above the heart to reduce blood pressure to the nose.

3. Lean forward so blood will pool in the nasal cavity, not run down the throat.

4. Use ice over the nose. (A bag of frozen peas is also excellent for this.)

5. If unsuccessful, place a piece of raw salt pork or bacon into the nostril, then apply pressure.

6. Repeat for up to 30 minutes, and if bleeding persists, seek emergency room care.

Any bleeding from any other orifice is significant with one exception. A small amount of blood on a toilet tissue after a bowel movement, or even drops of bright-red blood into the toilet, does not constitute an emergency but should be evaluated in a medical clinic. Bleeding from the bowel that continues for longer than a few minutes, vomiting blood, or copious blood from the rectum is reason to seek urgent care.

Spontaneous bleeding from the gums or uncontrolled bleeding from brushing your teeth or bleeding significantly out of proportion to the injury (hours of bleeding from a paper cut, for example) may be a sign of a blood or clotting disorder. This needs evaluation by a professional. If the bleeding can be stopped, it is not necessary to rush into an ER in the middle of the night, but do not wait more than the next day. The next bleed may be unstoppable.

INABILITY TO URINATE OR DEFECATE (HAVE A BOWEL MOVEMENT)

Sometimes if you are dehydrated, you may not void as normal, but sometimes there is a sudden blockage. Try taking clear liquids. If you cannot void at all or you feel your bladder or bowel is distending or "blowing up" in size, don't wait. This needs to be treated professionally and urgently. It may resolve spontaneously, but you still need to get it checked out.

Similarly, if you feel progressively bloated and cannot pass feces or gas, you may try drinking fluids, taking an enema, and/or drinking a laxative. If you have no luck getting gas to pass and feeling better, seek help. If you "decompress," you can wait until the morning, at least; but you need to be checked out. Significant bowel distention may be the harbinger of other diseases, such as cancer or infection or obstruction from an old surgical scar.

LESS SERIOUS CAUSES OF ABDOMINAL PAIN
Abdominal muscle strain
Dehydration
Diverticulitis
Food poisoning
Gallstones
Hernias
Indigestion
Irritable bowel syndrome
Kidney stones
Muscle hernia
Shingles
Urinary tract infection
Viral gastroenteritis with or w/o vomiting

ABDOMINAL PAIN

A certain abdominal tenderness or pain is to be expected if you have a flu-like illness and are vomiting. You can also pull an abdominal wall muscle. BUT persistent pain, especially localized to one area of the abdomen, abdominal pain accompanied by inability to pass gas or feces or urine, abdominal pain and fever—those conditions probably warrant a trip to the ER.

Today, when you are sick in any way, you have the luxury of running to a walk-in clinic or to a nearby ER to get a quick

MORE SERIOUS CAUSES

Angina or developing heart attack
Appendicitis
Hepatitis
Kidney infection
Obstruction from cancer
Obstruction from old surgery scarring
Pneumonia

check. In the future, when government-funded medicine causes even more shortages of manpower and facilities and gaps in emergency room availability, it is going to become a bigger hardship to access emergency care. Even now, waiting times in big-city emergency rooms may exceed six hours—even for people with chest pain! So it is important to start the search for emergency care early in the course of a problem. This chapter should have given you an idea of those medical situations in which you need to prepare for transport, and it should allow you to take appropriate measures before or while awaiting transport to higher-level care. In the next chapters, we will explore problems you can potentially completely care for at home without having to access scarce medical resources.

HOME REMEDIES FOR ABDOMINAL DISTENTION

- Add lemon and/or lime juice to water.

- Drink ginger, peppermint, licorice, or chamomile tea.

- Eat less food.

- Keep well hydrated with clear liquids.

- Maintain normal caffeine intake and add a little more.

- Stop smoking and drinking alcohol.

- Take a magnesium-containing laxative such as Milk of Magnesia. Also take 800 mg of MagCitrate daily.

- Take small amounts of baking soda.

18

WOUND MANAGEMENT

I n the course of our lives, we get wounded many times. Most wounds are minor and can be treated easily with a simple bandage. Sometimes they are more severe and require stitches. This chapter gives you a general approach and framework to think about wounds as surgeons do. When confronted with a wound, we automatically think through all the categories and put the wound into one. Then we look at the details and decide on a treatment strategy.

Evaluation: Wounds demand systematic evaluation and treatment. First, how was the wound made—in a clean environment? Or was it in a barnyard? How deep is the wound, and what structures are involved? Does it need suturing, or can it heal with lesser measures?

Environment: If the wound was contaminated with grease or road dirt or sand or any number of inorganic contaminants, it is at less risk of infection problems than if it was contaminated with organic material. Fecal material, such as horse manure or barnyard dirt, or mouth germs from bites need aggressive treatment.

What is injured? The best way to explore the wound without anesthesia is to evaluate function. In the hand, for example, can it move everything? Can it feel everything? Are pulses intact? After that, irrigate the wound with a normal saline solution made with one and a half teaspoons of salt in a pint of water. An ear bulb syringe is generally great for that. Use more than you think is necessary. Make sure the wound is really clean. Then look into the wound if it is deep. Small muscle lacerations don't need specific care; large ones do and will probably be beyond your ability to handle since they need sterile, deep-layered closure with a variety of sutures.

Butterfly bandage: Many small wounds can be cleansed and closed by pinching the skin together and sticking one or more Band-Aids or pieces of tape perpendicularly across the wound. In surgery we use tincture of benzoin to make the skin stickier, but degreasing with alcohol can work if you're careful not to pour it into the wound— that hurts! When you apply the sticky tape to close the wound, pinch the skin together enough so the skin edges "evert," or rise up a little, like buckled pavement. The reason for this is that when skin heals, it sinks in. If it starts totally flat, it will end a little depressed with a worse scar. In general the skin will need to be kept together for five to seven days. This does not work in any area where the skin is constantly stretched during motion (such as around the knee). This will pull the wound apart.

Suturing: Large, gaping wounds or wounds around knuckles or joints probably need suturing. Unless you are familiar with suturing, I would seek professional help. But as a surgeon, I keep a suture kit at home to avoid trips to the office or the ER. I sterilize the skin with alcohol and use a sterile towel to make a "sterile field" around the wound.

Leaving the wound open: Some wounds should not be closed—due to the high risk of infection. If in doubt, don't close it. The body has an amazing ability to shrink the size of wounds and to heal them with a much smaller scar than you would think. You can leave some part of the wound open for drainage, and close the clean ends with tape. The idea is not to trap bacteria behind a fixed, closed skin but to allow the body to expel the germs. Any wound previously closed that becomes infected should be opened, re-irrigated, and left open. Irrigate with the salt solution given previously and with a drop or two of antibiotic soap. Warm soaks in a tub three times a day are usually a good idea. Use the wet-to-dry dressing technique that follows. Wounds that have lost tissue and are like little craters should not be closed. Don't close anything you don't have to. Let the wisdom of the body do its work.

Antibiotics: Don't use antibiotics without a reason. For most small wounds, topical Neosporin or bacitracin ointment is sufficient. If you have a dirty wound or one of the aforementioned barnyard injuries, you may need to seek professional help. If you cannot, those involving significant tissue damage or fecal matter need aggressive early antibiotic administration. A combination of clindamycin (adult dose 300 milligrams three times a day) and cipro (adult dose 750 milligrams twice a day) covers most things. A friendly pharmacist may be able to give you good recommendations.

Dressings: Generally a dry dressing over a small amount of Neosporin is fine. If you need to care for a minor infection, a "wet to dry" dressing is useful.

For a wet-to-dry dressing, take standard gauze and pour onto the bandage some acetic acid solution (see sidebar). Wring out the gauze dressing as dry as possible and lay a single layer on the wound, avoiding much contact with normal skin. Cover with a dry dressing and an ACE wrap or a mesh encircling dressing.

1/4 PERCENT ACETIC ACID SOLUTION FOR WOUNDS
1 ounce white vinegar
15 ounces water
Add the vinegar to the water and mix well. Soak some gauze in the solution (usually 2 x 2-inch gauze pads work well). Wring out as much of the solution as possible so the gauze is only damp. Apply the moist gauze to the wound. Cover with a dry gauze dressing and secure with a circular wrap (preferable) or tape.

Healing Principles: There are several principles of healing that, if kept in mind, allow you to make good choices of care.

1. Skin heals best in moist, but not wet, settings.

2. Bacteria and infection slow healing.

3. Immobilization helps healing.

4. Good health and nutritional support are key to good healing.

Given these principles, if a cut keeps breaking open—say, on a finger—it is probably too dry. Add some Neosporin ointment to moisten. If a wound looks white and shriveled and is not healing, it is too wet. Open to air and/or use a dry dressing without ointment for a while. If a wound is at risk of infection or looks a little red, add antibiotic ointment. Big, scabby, road rashes that develop some superficial sliminess or obvious infection are well treated with an acetic acid wet-to-dry dressing in the morning and replaced with Neosporin and a dry dressing at night. And in all cases, vitamin C supplementation of a few thousand milligrams a day plus zinc supplementation of at least 60 milligrams a day have been shown to help wounds heal. If necessary, splint the area to avoid any stretching of the tissues.

Wound care is an art, and considerable experience and practice are needed to do it well. There are physicians whose entire specialization is taking care of difficult wounds. You cannot manage all wounds at home, but you will save yourself time, aggravation, and unnecessary trips to the ER if you understand the principles of wound care and can make good decisions about when you are able to care for the victim at home and when you need a higher level of care. Finally, it should be noted that wounds heal best in healthy people. Again, the best defense from the ravages of Obamacare on our medicine is to be so healthy you will not need care in the future.

19

RASHES

There is a joke in dermatology that it is not always necessary to make the diagnosis, just to make the right treatment. If it is wet—dry it. If it is dry—wet it, and otherwise apply cortisone or antifungal cream.

Most rashes are due to (1) allergic reaction, (2) fungus, (3) infection, or (4) insect bites. Without getting too technical, we are going to sort these out in a general way and give generalities of treatment. But the joke above is actually very true. If the treatment makes it worse—time to do the opposite. Common sense can go a long way in treating rashes.

ALLERGIC REACTION

Contact dermatitis: A very common "allergic" rash is contact dermatitis, in other words, an allergic response to having skin contact with a substance to which the body reacts. This can be poison ivy, or something as simple as your dish soap. Most such rashes are easy to figure out from the history and the distribution of the rash. If, for example, the rash is distributed in a nonrandom fashion (for example, occurring underneath elastic bands such as pajama waistbands, sock tops, or shirt sleeves)—voilà! It is either an allergy to the elastic or to something on the elastic, such as soap residue. It is important to know that healthy skin is less likely to react to contact with chemicals. But dry, cracked, or peeling skin can react more easily. Often, contact rashes occur when the skin is dry in the winter, but the same contact will not bother normal skin in the summer or spring.

If the rash seems to be related to clothing contact, it is time to look at your soap (any new soap?) and the quality of the skin. Make sure you use unscented laundry detergent without fillers. Avoid dryer sheets or any additive until you figure out the cause of the rash. You may have to eliminate everything then add things back one at a time. In the meantime, moisturize the skin with scent-free lotion, double rinse the clothes, and watch the rash over time. Do not use harsh soap on the body. Cetafil, if available, is the expensive dermatologist-recommended body wash you can get at a pharmacy. Homemade lye soap from olive oil and lard makes a beautiful mild soap. If you want to try your hand at making soap, you will find it easy, cheap, and great for nearly all skin types. See appendix C for my personal, easy-peasy soap recipe.

Contact dermatitis will usually respond to the measures just discussed, but you may sometimes need to apply hydrocortisone cream (0.5% to 1%) three times a day to the area for a few days until the rash clears. If it is getting worse, it may be a fungal rash (see below).

Hives: Hives are a very characteristic skin reaction to something contacted or ingested that causes the release of a chemical in the body called *histamine*. Hives are not just a skin problem. Of particular importance are hives in the mouth—these are more serious and require urgent medical intervention. Hives means you need to search for a cause. They can be the first sign of a more serious reaction involving facial, eyelid, and tongue swelling, and sometimes even airway compromise.

Hives are a raised, bumpy rash that is often spread far apart initially but becomes closer and closer. Hives sometimes produce a single sheet of raised, itchy, red skin. They can also "vesiculate" (become filled with clear fluid). This type of allergic reaction is "histamine mediated," so you generally start by taking an antihistamine. The most common over-the-counter one is probably Benadryl and should be taken orally as soon as possible. (Follow package directions.) This may cause drowsiness and should not be taken while driving or operating any heavy machinery. Topical cortisone cream may also help.

Once it is clear that the hives reaction is not progressing to a more serious allergic response, start looking for what caused them. Are the hives local or generalized? If local, did you come in contact with some nettles or poison ivy, some chemical, or perhaps latex?

If the response is generalized, look at medicines and food. Did you take a new medication within four or five hours of the event? Certain foods—egg whites being a common one—are more prone to causing this type of allergy. Seafood, especially shellfish, is a classic problem-producing allergen.

Eczema: Eczema is a rash classically produced by food allergies. It is a flat to slightly bumpy rash often involving the fronts of elbows, backs of knees, hands and feet, and occasionally the face. Sometimes the bumps can weep clear fluid when scratched, and it is very itchy. It is generally not rapidly progressive and can be figured out over time. Food allergies—especially eggs and milk—are likely culprits. But sometimes formal allergy testing is advised. I always recommend a gluten-free diet as a baseline.

FUNGUS

Skin rashes caused by fungus are common, the most common ones being jock itch, athlete's foot, and ringworm. Remember the old science experiment you probably did in grade school where you covered a slice of bread and left it in a dark place and it became green with mold? Skin fungus is similar in that it loves dark, moist places. So, jock itch happens in "sweaty" athletes, but it also happens in anyone who lets moisture stay trapped under clothing for prolonged periods. Fungal rashes occur under clothing and in areas of skin folds primarily. Certain things, like a T-shirt under clothing that traps moisture, can cause ringworm to develop in the chest area.

These rashes are flat and red and, in the case of ringworm, have a characteristic circular ring. Candida (another common fungus) rashes have red, flat, itchy spots with a spreading edge of tiny little "satellite" lesions.

As noted earlier, rashes caused by fungus respond rapidly to a good antifungal over-the-counter cream. In addition, it is important to avoid moisture trapping. Remove T-shirts and wear blousy clothing. After showering, dry areas of skin folds with a towel and/or blow dryer, being careful to dry thoroughly under breasts, in the groin, between toes, and between butt cheeks. (Painful cracking between buttock cheeks may be a sign of a fungal rash.)

INFECTION

Cellulitis is not a "rash" but presents as red, sometimes itchy skin. Cellulitis is an infection in the skin, usually spreading from some source of the infection such as a splinter or wound. This is generalized redness over an area (not spots) and may be painful and tender. Cellulitis is usually flat and may be streaking, and it is almost always warm to the touch. Cellulitis should send you to the doctor. But if no immediate care is available, look for and remove the source (a splinter, for example), and start antibiotics as previously discussed. Cipro and clindamycin are a good choice. Soak open wounds in warm water. Then try to get help because these things can go bad quickly.

INSECT BITES

Sometimes multiple insect bites can mimic a rash, but technically these are a different thing altogether. The most common bite "rash" comes from *chiggers*—tiny little insects that get into the waistband of your pants or the tops of socks while you are working outside in grasslands or woodlands. These bites are terribly itchy but resolve without much of a problem. If you need treatment, calamine lotion or topical cortisone is usually effective. Fleas and bedbugs should be suspected if the problem is ongoing. Fleas you can usually see eventually, but bedbugs are often invisible except in the mattress. Bedbugs may give a regional rash and may persist because of continued biting.

As mentioned earlier, new diseases are being introduced into the United States with the illegal immigrant population. One such disease is malaria, a disease spread to humans from mosquito bites. Surprising to some, malaria was once endemic (common) in the Midwest at the time of the pioneers. The more human carriers of malaria, the more chance of mosquitos acquiring the parasite from a human bite and then spreading it to the next victim. To prevent infection from biting insects, you must know their habits, wear appropriate clothing, and use an effective bug spray. For mosquitos, avoid being out at dusk, wear a long-sleeved shirt when possible, and use an effective repellant as indicated. Repellants containing Deet are usually effective against mosquitoes.

20

COLDS AND FLU-LIKE ILLNESSES

t is common for every viral illness to be called "the flu." But in reality, "flu" is one specific disease caused by a family of viruses called *influenza*. Most colds and flu-like illnesses are not influenza but, rather, are caused by a host of less serious but annoying viruses that give us the well-known symptoms of running nose, itchy eyes, achiness, fever, and sometimes nausea and vomiting. Food poisoning—food contaminated with bacteria—is probably the most common reason for diarrhea and vomiting, especially when those symptoms occur together. But food poisoning is often misdiagnosed by both patients and doctors as "flu." Here are some specifics on the various culprits that make you feel sick:

Colds: A cold is annoying to miserable but generally not serious. The major problem is disruption of sleep and productivity. Symptoms of a common cold are well known to most people—runny and/or stuffy nose; runny, itchy, or burning eyes; feverishness; sore throat; fatigue; and sometimes chills.

Treatment for most colds consists of making the symptoms better. Since colds are caused by viruses and antibiotics do not treat viruses, we do *not* use antibiotics for the common cold. Unwarranted use of antibiotics can cause a person to develop an immunity to antibiotics, and this can limit options later in life when more serious illnesses may hit.

Treatment is generally rest, keeping warm, taking fluids, avoiding alcohol, and giving the cold time to resolve. Although it is controversial in standard medicine, many in the anti-aging community[1] believe in high-dose vitamin C for treating acute cold symptoms. Years ago, I was in a busy spinal surgery practice with a high overhead that didn't stop when I got sick. I developed a bad cold with all the classic symptoms, including a terrible runny nose and fatigue. But I had a full OR schedule the next day. (It is tough to operate with a nose running into your surgical mask; trust me.) So I went to my nurse friend and asked her to plug me into an IV that I supplied, containing 50,000 milligrams of vitamin C. This is a very high dose—the usual tablet being 250 to 1,000 milligrams. But I had read and heard about this protocol at an anti-aging meeting and decided to give it a try. My friend was dubious at best, but I assured her I would not hold her responsible for the outcome! She plugged me in to the IV as I sat at her kitchen counter with a red runny nose, runny eyes, feverishness, and chills. During the hour it took to run in the liter of vitamin C fluid, we sat at the counter and chatted. She told me at the end of the hour that she could actually see me getting better by the minute, as the redness in my nose faded before her eyes. My eyes stopped watering, and I felt about 80 percent better. I was fine by the next morning and was able to finish my surgery day. Placebo effect? I don't think so, because so many docs have had similar experiences with themselves or their patients. Since then I have kept IV supplies and large-dose vitamin C in my office for desperate times.

Now, you won't have the ability to plug into IV vitamin C, but you can boost your levels by taking vitamin C orally. However, you cannot take massive amounts of vitamin C orally without getting diarrhea, so the best option is to take 1,000 milligrams every hour or hour and a half. The minute you feel any loose bowel movement coming on, back off. In lesser cases of cold-like symptoms, I do just this: at the first sign of a cold, I start taking 1,000 milligrams every hour for a few hours, then every hour and a half.

As noted earlier, don't take Tylenol and don't take any anti-inflammatory to lower your temperature or treat achiness. The body has a well-developed system for fighting infection. When a viral or bacterial invader is discovered, the immune system cells that encounter the germs send out a chemical alert to call for help in fighting the invaders. Just as in war, the front-line troops (in this case white cells) hold the invader at bay, sacrificing themselves in the process, while calling for reinforcements. Through chemical signaling with "cytokines," these cells have called for other cells to join them. When enough invaders are present and a big response is required, the front-line troop cells send out so many cytokines that we refer to it as a "cytokine storm." A cytokine storm is a normal, healthy response to invading organisms. When we use chemicals to lower the temperature, we disrupt this signaling mechanism. Sponging, or applying a cool T-shirt and other nonmedicinal means, physically lowers the temperature but does not impair the body's immune signaling. Even so, I do not recommend decreasing a fever unless it is over 104 degrees or very uncomfortable. Usually temperature is not a predominant complaint with the common cold.

The cold symptom that makes me most miserable is a stuffy nose and inability to breathe at night. I like using a nasal spray, like Afrin, spritzing a little into each nostril at bedtime. But do this only for three days, as prolonged use of Afrin or its generic counterparts can cause damage to your nose from over-constriction of the blood vessels.

An antihistamine such as Zyrtec or Claritin—or my favorite OTC antihistamine, cetirizine—really helps runny noses and the itchy-eye problem. These second-generation drugs tend to be less sedating than, say, Benadryl. But at nighttime you may want the Benadryl. I tend to stay away from liquid combination cold remedies because many contain Tylenol.

And "forcing fluids"—making yourself drink fruit juice, water, watery soup, even soda pop—when you would rather just lie there, makes sense. The curative power of chicken soup may be just an old wives' tale, but it sure seems to be what the body wants during a cold. As they say, "Feed a cold, starve a fever." In recent years, kale seems to have become the fashionable veggie, and during a cold this year, my hospital administrator gave me kale vegetable soup. It sure seemed to turn the tide of the illness, and it tasted just like what my body needed. I believe in listening to the body.

As a preventive measure, I make sure to take high-dose vitamin D—10,000 units a day to boost my immune system. Also I take at least 1,000 milligrams (1 gram) of vitamin C a day. I love the GNC version of chewable C from rose hips. It just flat-out tastes good and can be chewed without gagging. And I keep vitamin C at my office computer so I can chew some regularly if I am exposed to someone with a cold. When I have a cold or any illness, I take 1,000 milligrams of vitamin C every couple of hours while awake.

There is an over-the-counter nutriceutical called Epicor, which I believe helps decrease all such illness. The drug was developed in Iowa by a farmer who created it for his cattle. With it, he was able to decrease the stillbirths and improve the health of his herds of both beef cattle and pigs. His homemade fermentation became so popular among the farmers in his area that he gave up farming and went into full-time production. His company grew, and his business split into a factory building and an administrative building. Some years later, when health care and insurance got more complicated and expensive, he hired a firm to set up a self-insurance program. In running their actuarial studies, they noticed that those employees who worked in the factory never got sick or took any sick days. But the employees in the administration building got sick as usual. Furthermore, if a person from admin went to work in the factory, after about three months he or she no longer had sick days, and vice versa: people going from the factor to the admin building were good for about three months, then they started getting minor illness and took time off from work. It caused them to really study the product the farmer had created. It turns out that the product doesn't directly kill germs or directly affect white cells. But if you think of the body's immune system as an orchestra with many different instruments, Epicor somehow acts like an orchestra conductor, optimizing how the immune system components work together.

So what do I do? I take 10,000 IU of vitamin D a day, 1,000 IU of vitamin C a day when not sick, and one tablet of Epicor a day. Although I have been sick and although it is good to challenge our immune systems occasionally, since doing all this I rarely get colds or flu-like illnesses as I did in the past. And the same is true of my patients on the same anti-aging regimen. A controlled study? No. Convincing in my clinical practice? You bet. Ultimately you can choose.

Influenza: Sometimes things start out as "colds" but ultimately manifest as something else. True influenza may begin with cold-like symptoms but develops a different constellation of symptoms with time, including higher fevers—up to 105 degrees—chills, and more severe malaise (tiredness, achiness, and a general feeling of being unwell). The fever may come and go. Muscle aches and pains may be prominent. You may have headache and photophobia (light bothering your eyes). Some people progress to pneumonia, but this is rare. (It was a rapidly fatal pneumonia that resulted in the deaths during the pandemic of 1918 that killed millions.) True influenza can last up to two weeks. The treatment for influenza without any complications (see next section) is the same as for the common cold, with one exception. You may need to take measures to lower your temperature if you are quite miserable, but don't do it with pills. Instead, you can sit in a bathtub and sponge down with tepid water, or you can put on a T-shirt soaked in warm water, then let it cool off in the room air while you are lying in bed. I have found that very effective.

Complications: Complications of a cold or flu are usually "superimposed infections"—pneumonia, bronchitis, or sinusitis. You may start with a runny nose that plugs your sinus passages. Then bacteria colonize the backed-up nasal secretions, and the next thing you know, you are blowing out yellow or greenish slime from your nose. That is the hallmark of bacteria taking over an otherwise viral illness. Although antibiotics don't help the viral part, they will help clear the bacterial infection. Similarly, a cough that was producing clear mucus may begin producing phlegm that is colored yellow or brownish. In these cases you need treatment with antibiotics and should seek medical care. These infections need to be completely cleared, and this takes more than a few days of antibiotics. You need a full course of meds and supervision. Generally, we treat from five to ten days depending on the severity of the illness and the strength of the antibiotic chosen.

Of course, any infection that causes throat swelling and airway compromise is a flat-out emergency.

Food poisoning: Since food poisoning can be misunderstood to be flu, we will address the symptoms here. True influenza with gastrointestinal symptoms lasts for more than a few days, generally causes diarrhea, but rarely causes a sudden onset of vomiting and diarrhea all at once. Sudden onset of abdominal bloating, diarrhea, nausea, and vomiting that lasts a day or less is generally food poisoning. Depending on the bacteria involved, it may start two to sixteen hours or more after ingestion of the contaminated food. You can look for a source—my husband was clearly poisoned by an egg salad sandwich in an airport once—but usually the source is unclear. In the absence of dysentery (bloody diarrhea), you just keep replacing fluids and let it resolve. If you have true dysentery, seek help and be cautious not to contaminate others. Scrupulous hand washing and isolation from family members, if possible, may prevent its spreading.

LIFE STAGE GROUP	NIH RECOMMENDATIONS VITAMIN D RDA (IU / DAY)	DR. HIEB'S RECOMMENDATIONS VITAMIN C (MG / DAY)	VITAMIN D RDA (IU / DAY)	VITAMIN C (MG / DAY)
INFANTS 0–6 MONTHS	*	40		
INFANTS 6–12 MONTHS	*	50		
1–3 YEARS OLD	*	15	1,000	500
4–8 YEARS OLD	600	25	5,000	500
9–13 YEARS OLD	600	45	5,000	1,000
14–18 YEARS OLD	600	65	10,000	AT LEAST 1,000
14–18 YEARS OLD, PREGNANT / LACTATING	600	115	10,000	AT LEAST 1,000
19–30 YEARS OLD	600	90	10,000	AT LEAST 1,000
19–50 YEARS OLD, PREGNANT / LACTATING	600	120	10,000	AT LEAST 1,000
31–50 YEARS OLD	600	75	10,000	AT LEAST 1,000
51–70 YEARS OLD (MALES)	600	80	10,000	AT LEAST 1,000
51–70 YEARS OLD (FEMALES)	600	80	10,000	AT LEAST 1,000
71+ YEARS OLD	800		10,000	AT LEAST 1,000

*For infants, adequate intake is 400 IU/day for 0 to 6 months of age and 400 IU/day for 6 to 12 months of age.[1]

As a cynical observation, I have noted in medicine that the more treatments we have for a problem, the less successful any of the treatments are in actually solving the problem. In the past we had 105 procedures to correct bunion deformity of the feet. (I think—I hope—we are doing better in the past twenty years.) Jesus said, "You will always have the poor among you" (John 12:8

NIV). Hippocrates should have said, "You will always get colds; just live with it." You will not avoid colds, and it is probably beneficial to get the occasional flu or flu-like illness, as it keeps your immune system in shape.

The question is what can we do to alleviate the misery from these colds that always hit at the worst possible time? Well, it is always good to get advice from a doctor who has your disease. I have had a lot of colds in my life, and I've told you all I know to do for my family and myself. I cannot emphasize enough the benefit of vitamin D_3. This vitamin is one of the most powerful anti-aging and disease-protecting substances we have in our medical arsenal. Take it. Take it in big doses. Do not believe the government doses, which are based on no evidence. (In the anti-aging world we refer to the RDA as the "Recommended Death Allowance.") And take vitamin C. Eat a good diet, get enough sleep, and exercise as outlined in chapter 8. Taken together, all of this will cut down—but not eliminate—the episodes of colds and flu you experience.

21

BITES

We talked about bites briefly in previous chapters, but in this chapter we will cover them in more depth.

Bite wounds are pretty straightforward. One thing, however, is unique and should be kept in mind. Bites cause swelling. It is tempting to apply ice to a bite wound to prevent swelling, but DON'T APPLY ICE. It turns out that cold activates many venoms and quite probably will make the situation worse. If you lump all kinds of bites together, there are only three treatment types: *symptomatic therapy, surgery and antibiotics,* or *antivenom.*

Common insect bites: Most insect bites require only symptomatic treatment. Use calamine lotion for itching, keeping the area clean and moisturizing as needed. Dry skin is always more susceptible to itching and scaling, and dry skin generally worsens any problem.

Tick bites: Ticks are annoying and are becoming more of a problem because of Lyme disease. Most ticks that get on people are "wood ticks," or the American dog tick—the flat, brown bug with black highlights that is generally about two to four millimeters in size. These do not generally carry Lyme disease, but all ticks can carry some type of a tick-borne illness, such as Rocky Mountain spotted fever. The classic wood tick is easily visible, whereas the deer tick, most classically associated with Lyme disease, may be so small it is missed.

If you have a tick attached to you, the classic removal technique is to heat the tick's body with a hot pin or other source of focal heat. This causes the tick to start backing out or releasing its grip, and you can then remove it without losing the head within the skin.

The most important point is to monitor for any symptoms that occur after the bite: a round, red rash, flu-like illness, joint aches and pains, or any systemic illness occurring within weeks of the bite should receive prompt treatment. Classically, doxycycline 100 milligrams twice a day for ten to twenty-one days is prescribed. It is important not to let your doctor minimize the symptoms as unrelated because, if the doctor is wrong, long-term arthritic symptoms can set in. It is better to be overcautious and treat rather than withhold treatment for absolute proof—which is never available because lab studies are notorious for missing the early disease.

Spider bites: Most spider bites just need local care and time to go away—they are simply annoying. If you see the spider, capture it and hold it in a container in case you develop symptoms. Symptoms of a black widow spider bite begin within an hour and are systemic—nausea, shaking, numbness, pain, and flu-like illness: muscle cramps, abdominal pain, and so forth. A brown recluse bite may go unnoticed at first because the bites are not always painful. But over hours the wound becomes painful and red, and over days, death of the tissue around the bite may occur. In short, if you suspect either of these bites, go to an emergency room. These need aggressive medical care. There is no home treatment. Do not apply ice. Support the victim with hydration and protection and warmth if needed.

These venomous species—black widows and brown recluse spiders—are not aggressive. They hide in warm, dry places. They are very prevalent in the desert areas of America and love things such as cardboard boxes.[1] During my many military moves, I lived in the desert and had partially unpacked cardboard boxes in the garage, which had been colonized by black widows. I occasionally found black widows taking up residence in some of my houseplants. When I found them in the house, I removed them. But I know that we didn't find them all, and we lived for years in a communal arrangement where I instructed my children not to reach into dark places or into my houseplants without observing for spiders. (In those days we also had a house gecko living in our couch, and he only came out during spring cleaning!)

Snake Bites: North Carolina has every species of poisonous snake, and there are by far more envenomations in North Carolina than in any other state in the union. As a surgeon, I took care of United States Marine Corps members for years in North Carolina. These Marines made a living snooping and crawling through hot, humid forests. Nevertheless, most snake bites were the result of doing something demonstrably (and sometimes catastrophically) stupid. In short, if you don't reach blindly into your woodpile or other areas where snakes go to get out of the sun, if you don't try to be Bear Grylls by capturing a snake and biting its head off (yes, young men really do that), if you wear tall boots through the brush, and if you learn to make noise before going through grasslands and other areas where snakes live—you probably won't get bitten. If you do, and you can observe the snake, do so. Don't try to capture a snake. Venomous snakes in the United States have triangular heads and either diamond patterns or bright rings (coral snake) and often rattles.

Not all snakebites are envenomations, but don't take chances. If bitten, don't ice the wound, and don't cut and suck the wound. Head to the nearest emergency room. You cannot take a chance on waiting. Go immediately. (See chapter 17, "Real Emergencies That Can't Wait.") Unfortunately, the treatment for envenomation is—as we say in orthopaedics—"antivenom, antivenom, antivenom." If Obamacare pushes us to single-party payer or we experience overall system collapse, antivenom may not be available everywhere, and in these cases we may be simply out of luck.

Bee/Wasp Stings: Bees can sting you only once, and then they die. In the absence of an allergy to bee stings, this is annoying but not life-threatening. The stinger gets deposited in your skin and is generally easily removed by carefully scratching it with your nail or a knife. Do not attempt to grasp the stinger, as that may inject more poison into you. An exception would be a mass stinging because bee venom is toxic to the heart in big enough doses. If you experience a mass stinging, get professional help.

I used to be a beekeeper. One day I failed to secure my bee helmet and netting, and there was a small hole where the net contacted the chest. As I was working the hive, a single bee penetrated my hood and began to sting me on the inside of my left nostril. Now, had I simply reflected upon the fact that the bee could sting me only once and had I quietly walked away, all would have been well. But to be honest, it is hard to be calm and collected when a bee is in your nose. So I reflexively lunged for my face and knocked the whole hood apparatus off. Sensing opportunity, hundreds of bees swarmed out to defend the hive, bearing down on my face and long hair, which had come tumbling out. I ran into the dark basement, screaming as my husband laughed himself silly. (Running into the dark works for the average Italian honeybee, but an Africanized bee may chase you for miles through dark and light.) In the basement, my head was abuzz with bees trapped in my hair. My husband finally collected himself enough to help me by getting a hairbrush and getting rid of the bees. By that time, of course, I probably had been stung more than fifteen times. Initially, I experienced stinging and some facial swelling, but the excitement came twelve hours later as I lay in bed and became lightheaded. I felt more and more as if I would black out, and I could not detect my own pulse. I took deep breaths and raised my legs above my heart. But, nothing changed. My husband tried to call an ambulance, but in those days there was no 911 where we lived and the phone line was busy. Fortunately, I just had a touch of asthma—probably from being allergic to the many flowers in my yard—and I kept an Alupent inhaler at the bedside. The drug in the inhaler causes the heart to speed up, and after I took a few puffs, my heart rate recovered, and I felt fine. I called my friendly cardiologist, and he had no clue about this phenomenon after bee stings. But my friend who was both an anesthesiologist and a beekeeper knew about the slowing of the heart that can occur with a large injection of bee venom. In fact, this is what can kill you when swarms of Africanized bees attack you—even if you are not allergic to bee stings.

If you are allergic to bee stings, of course, keep an EpiPen on you or nearby at all times, and know how to use it.

Everything we just covered also applies to wasp stings—except that these little guys can sting you and sting you again! Wasps don't lose their stingers in you so the right response is to get the heck out of their nest area.

Human and animal bites: See the chapter on "Real Emergencies That Can't Wait" for more information, but in general, you treat these with cleansing, antibiotic ointment, and observation. But be aware that human and animal bites can become infected with exotic bad germs. At the first sign of trouble, seek medical attention. Generally, it is safer not to close these wounds. If a human bite starts looking red, hot, and swollen and you have no immediate medical assistance available, make sure the wound can drain. If necessary, remove any scabbing or reopen the skin margins. Soak the affected area in a warm sink or tub of water, or by placing a moist warm towel on the area. It is even possible to apply a moist cloth and cover it with a heating pad. The point is to keep moisture on the wound and to keep the blood flow stimulated with warmth. Apply an antibiotic ointment and alternate with ¼ percent acetic acid wet-to-dry dressing changes as outlined on page 185. Clean daily with soap and water as well. Take 750 milligram cipro every twelve hours and 300 milligram clindamycin by mouth three times a day. For children use Clindamicin 30 mg/kg per day, divided into three doses. (See sidebar on page 168.)

Bite wounds are like the practice of anesthesia—usually boring, but occasionally things happen to set your hair on fire, and you have to act quickly and appropriately. I hope medical care will always be available, but sadly, the first things to become scarce in a socialist health care model like Obamacare are expensive medications and those items used only occasionally. Antivenom is one such item. Jeffrey Tucker of the Mises Institute gives a very funny talk about our current regulatory environment. He points out that the sanitation of flushing away human waste has been improving for nearly five hundred years since the first flushing systems. But the government, via the EPA, has managed in five years to give us toilets that don't succeed at their primary function—flushing away human waste. In medicine, the more serious consequences of our overregulation will be unnecessary death as antivenom, trauma surgeons, and emergency rooms are in shorter and shorter supply.

22

SPRAINS, STRAINS, AND BROKEN BONES

B y definition a *sprain* is stretching and/or tearing of a liga-
ment—a fibrous band connecting bone to bone. A *strain* is
either a muscle injury or injury to the tendon that connects
muscle to bone. Broken bones are *fractures*.

SPRAINS

Sprains generally involve the ankle or wrist and are caused by twisting
or overextending the joint. There is swelling and tenderness over the
soft tissue of the ligaments, and sometimes bruising will be noticed
later. The only way to completely rule out a fracture is an X-ray, but
the following rules generally apply. You can probably watch and wait
unless you have the triad of bone tenderness, focal swelling, and
bruising over the area of tenderness. These indicate a fracture.

Initial treatment consists of elevating the extremity, applying ice
to the area, and splinting if possible. Usually a sprain will be much
better in seventy-two hours, but total healing time is longer, so don't
expect *complete* resolution.

An exception to all this is a knee sprain. Knee ligaments are
extremely important and unforgiving. A twisting injury to the knee

that results in swelling needs professional orthopaedic evaluation—not in the middle of the night but as soon as practicable.

SPLINT AMAL

- ❏ An arm sling
- ❏ Moldable splint material (you can order A + Z Medical Professional Emergency Veterinary Splint on Amazon for around $14)
- ❏ An "air cast" splint for ankle sprains
- ❏ One-inch silk tape and 2 x 2-inch gauze for buddy taping
- ❏ Several (3- and 4-inch) ACE wraps

When applying splints, there are certain principles: Always apply a splint over cloth, a sock, or an ACE wrap. Never splint directly on the skin, as this may cause blistering and skin death. Try to splint an extremity in as close to a normal use position as possible. Don't splint fingers if the wrist is all that is involved. Stiffness is the biggest problem with prolonged splinting. If you are going to watch and see, you should rest, ice, and observe for seventy-two hours, and then remove the splint and reassess. Never use a too-tight ACE wrap. Remove the splint if there is any increasing numbness, tingling, or pain. If pain becomes unbearable, something is wrong—usually the swelling is compressing nerves or blood supply, and this needs immediate emergency room attention.

If you dislocate and relocate a finger, you can buddy tape it to a neighboring finger and seek orthopaedic care during the light of day. To buddy tape, put dry two-by-two-inch gauze between the fingers, then lay the tape around the two fingers at two points: above the joint and below the joint. Just lay the tape on; don't stretch it or make it too tight.

All fractures that are not open and are generally aligned can be splinted and seen in an orthopaedic office within forty-eight hours. Even the slightest pinhole around the fracture is an emergency. All dislocations, open fractures, severely angulated fractures, or fractures with any nerve or circulation compromise need urgent professional care.

HOW TO WRAP A SPLINT USING A SAM SPLINT

DOUBLE LAYER WRIST

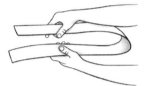

Step 1: Fold a 36-inch SAM Splint in half upon itself.

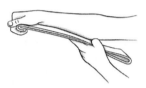

Step 2: Roll the end over to provide more comfort for the fingers.

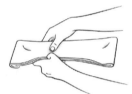

Step 3: Add strength by creating a C curve.

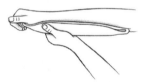

Step 4: Using your own arm as a template, mold the splint to the general shape of the wrist and forearm.

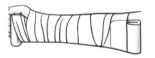

Step 5: Make adjustments to fit the injury and apply to the patient. Only small adjustments should be made once the splint is in place. Secure with your wrap of choice.

ANKLE STIRRUP

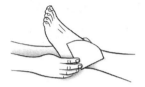

Step 1: If footwear is removed or when the ankle is exposed, place padding above and around the boney prominences on each side of the ankle.

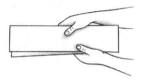

Step 2: Fold a 36-inch SAM Splint to create two equal halves.

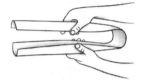

Step 3: Apply C curves two-thirds of the distance down each half. Add reverse C curves on the edges if needed for strength. Do not extend the curves further or they will stiffen the splint and limit your ability to fold it around the foot or ankle.

Step 4: Fold the stirrup splint around the foot and ankle.

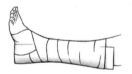

Step 5: Secure with your wrap of choice.

In concluding this chapter, as an orthopaedic surgeon, I cannot resist recounting a little history.

"Bone setting" is an ancient practice described in the oldest extant medical text—the Edwin Smith papyrus from Egypt, dated around 1500 BC. Although straightening and splinting fractures and dislocations uses very commonsense principles, the actual techniques have always required dexterity, experience, and skill. "Bonesetters" have always been a bit separate from the rest of medicine. Sometimes fracture care was done by barber-surgeons, but it was never practiced by "true" physicians. Friendly rivalry between internal medicine physicians and orthopaedists still exists. In primitive cultures the local witch doctor may have set bones, or he subcontracted to a specialist who did nothing but bone setting. Today, in spite of the spread of Western medicine generally, this practice continues in sub-Saharan Africa, where (as in Nigeria) nearly 85 percent of fracture care is rendered by traditional unlicensed "bonesetters."

23

BACK AND NECK PAIN

I keep a copy of a Gahan Wilson cartoon framed on my wall. In it, a patient is sitting on an examination table with his shirt off, and there is an ugly green lizard-like beast clinging to the patient's back. The doctor, poking at the beastie with his finger, says, "Mr. Jones, I believe we've found the source of your back pain." Although the cartoon is humorous, it brings up an important point: thorough clinical examination is a key component of diagnostic medicine. In today's world of government-run health care, lesser-trained medical providers are replacing doctors, and all of us are being overwhelmed with computer work that takes time away from patient care. Careful physical examination is often skipped over. Many patients tell me, a spinal surgeon, that after going from doctor to doctor, I am the first one to actually have them undress and examine the back. But that is important because not all back pain is caused by spinal injury. I haven't found a green lizard, but I have found a number of shingles rashes, and shingles will cause several weeks of back pain before it resolves. I have also found burns from heating pads, wallets that are too big to sit on repeatedly without compressing the sciatic nerve, and marks from too-heavy backpacks or overweighted police duty belts.

So all back pain is not from the spine. If your back pain is associated with vomiting, illness, alteration of bowel habits, and so forth, seek medical help. This chapter is for treatment of the everyday, garden-variety back pain.

Back pain is commonly due to an insult to the little joints in our spines or our disks—the hydraulic shock absorbers that separate the spinal bones. It is a popular misconception that back pain is muscular. Usually it is not. Muscle spasm is a secondary phenomenon caused by joint irritation.

The usual story goes something like this: "I was helping move furniture [or other objects] over a period of several hours. My back didn't hurt right away, but later that night I started to have low back pain. By morning I could barely move. Any motion hurts, but its better when I lie down."

This is the classic "overuse" syndrome. The little joints in the back get abused, so they swell and hurt. Usually this kind of back pain is better but not totally gone in three days. Treatment consists of rest; anti-inflammatories, such as Naproxen (440–500 mg, twice a day); a hot pack or ice to the area (whichever feels better); and time to resolve. You can stretch the lower back by lying on the floor with your legs over a chair or the couch seat and then bringing your knees slowly to your chest. Hold for ten seconds; then return to the starting position. Relax for thirty seconds, and then repeat the exercise a few times. Take the Naproxen every day until several days *after* you stop having pain, to prevent recurrence.

Disk injury: A disk injury may start off just as the back pain did in the hypothetical furniture-moving case. Or it may occur with a sudden lifting, twisting injury, or with very little trauma at all. These disk problems usually occur in people over thirty who have done "daily microtrauma" to their disks by repeated bending, causing small cracks to occur in the outside elastic ring of the disk. These cracks eventually form a channel. Through this channel of cracks, the inside jelly part of the disk "herniates" into the outside of the disk, giving you horrible back pain that can last for two to three weeks. Sometimes, the interior jelly material pushes *completely* outside of the disk, lodging next to the nerve that goes down your buttock and leg. This can give you the classic symptoms of *sciatica*—buttock and/or leg pain, burning, numbness, and worsening of pain with sitting or bending. You may also have some foot weakness. The treatment for disk damage is initially the same as for other back pain—rest, Naproxen, and time. This will take longer, usually two to three weeks. And total healing of the disk occurs over two years. To allow the channel to seal over and heal, it is important not to pressurize the disk by sitting, lifting, or forward bending. In general your activities at first should be limited to walking and standing or lying down. For at least two weeks, avoid sitting or bending. Take the Naproxen faithfully until the pain is gone for at least a week or two. If at any time you have progressive weakness, any inability to void, numbness in the groin area, loss of erectile function, or bowel incontinence—seek emergency help.

Of note, smoking is a leading cause of disk disease because one cigarette closes down the blood supply to the disk by 50 percent for twelve hours. So, your disks do not have the ability to heal themselves between episodes of use. To keep your back healthy, don't smoke, stay thin, avoid repeated bending, and keep your core muscles in good shape.

Neck pain: The principles for avoiding and treating back pain are generally true for neck pain too. Most neck pain is due to a lifetime of repeatedly looking down, flexing our necks. We were designed to be hunter-gatherers, spending most of our days looking out over the plains in search of game. Our heads were balanced on our torsos, and the little "rocker bearing" joints didn't get overused. But today our civilized selves spend hours a day looking down at schoolbooks (or at a surgical patient), or we sit reading in bed with our necks too flexed. If you have neck pain, do as I recommended for the back. Rest the neck in a neutral, non-flexed position, take

Naproxen, and give it time. If arm pain or weakness develops and is progressive, seek help.

To prevent problems with your neck, avoid a prolonged flexed position. Don't sleep on too big a pillow. Your neck and head need to be straight with the torso. Use a small, squishy, down pillow or a rolled-up towel. (The towel is helpful in avoiding neck pain in hotel rooms from those too-big, pretty pillows.) Don't read without elevating your book. Dittos for knitting or other activities you might do in your bed. Put a pillow under your arms and raise up your work. On an airplane put that pillow under your lower back, not your head. Practice good posture, keeping your head balanced, like a ballerina, over your body.

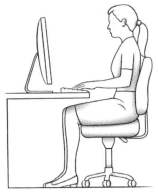

good posture at a desk

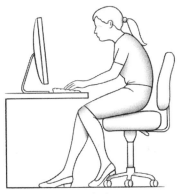

bad posture at a desk

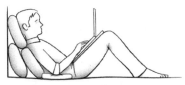

good posture in bed

bad posture in bed

I could make a living off people who work in front of a computer and the neck pain they suffer. Get your keyboard up so that, when you're keyboarding, your arms are at 90 degrees elbow flexion and you are generally looking straight ahead or up a little. The worst ergonomic thing ever invented was that little pullout keyboard that is nearly on your lap, forcing you to look down all day. Don't use those. If necessary, put those out-of-date books under your laptop to elevate it.

Upper back pain: Less commonly, someone will reach for an object above chest level and experience a sudden sharp pain in the upper back. You can do the self-treatments outlined earlier, but if this pain is not resolved in twenty-four hours, consider a visit to the chiropractor. I've found chiropractic manipulation is extremely helpful in solving this problem in short order. Unfortunately, if the pain sets in over weeks, it is then hard to treat successfully to resolution.

In each of my examination rooms I have a framed copy on the wall of my rules for a healthy back.

DR. HIEB'S RULES FOR A HEALTHY BACK

1. **Don't smoke.** Smoking kills bone cells and decreases oxygen to the disks.

2. **Stay thin.** Every extra pound in abdominal weight translates to several pounds of added pressure to disks.

3. **Choose to be happy.** Victor Frankl learned in Auschwitz that we cannot always choose what happens to us but we can choose how we react. It does not help to focus on things we cannot change. Sometimes we have to live with arthritic back pain. I cannot sit on the floor with my children the way I could when I was younger. Some back pain is a fact of life, and rather than become debilitated, we should do what we can to be fulfilled in life and to reach out to others.

---

4. **Be physically fit.** Core strength is key to improving and avoiding back pain.

5. **Use good back mechanics.** Avoid twisting, bending, and leaning.

6. **Think ergonomically.** Use your head, not your back. Find back-safe ways of doing the job.

7. **Avoid reinjury.** When that air conditioner you just bought starts to fall off the truck—ya gotta let it go. Choose to save your back, not the replaceable object.

24

FOOT PAIN

Foot pain is either focal (involving one discrete spot), in a bigger area over the mid-foot, or localized to the arch, the heel, or the "ball" of the foot. A lot of foot pain is due to shoe wear, so you should not try to squeeze your feet into too-narrow shoes. The best shoes for your feet have a wide toe box and good crepe soles and are built for the activity you are doing. Don't play tennis in running shoes, and vice versa. As you get older, your feet need more padding; avoid standing barefoot, and wear well-padded shoes as much as possible. Another thing, which is not talked about in the literature but which is very clear from my practice, is the association of hormone loss with foot pain. When women go through menopause, they commonly develop foot pain—stiffness in the morning and pain with prolonged standing. This usually resolves with appropriate hormone therapy.

Focal pain is pain that is especially localized under the balls of the feet and is usually due to aging and loss of fat padding. Insoles may help this, or you can place a pad just behind the balls of the feet to take the pressure off the bony prominences under the ball of the foot. Some local pain is due to corns or calluses that become enlarged and thickened and become pressure points. You can trim these with a toenail clipper (or scalpel blade, to be traditional). Check for abnormal shoe pressure that may be causing this.

Heel pain that is under the heel proper (calcaneal bursitis) or at the junction of the heel and the arch (plantar fasciitis) can be a nuisance and may take time to resolve. Treatment consists of anti-inflammatories, weight loss if obese, and plastic heel cups that squeeze the heel while walking. This effectively gives you more heel padding.

Mid-arch pain is in the mid-foot and is worse in the morning, gets better after a little walking, but gets worse again after a lot of walking. It is classic arthritis pain. The treatment includes good shoes, avoiding going barefoot, choosing a sport other than walking or running for exercise, and taking Naproxen or other anti-inflammatory as needed.

Toe pain: In the absence of deformity, pain in the toes can be pressure from shoe wear, commonly called a "Morton's neuroma." Morton's neuroma is compression of the nerves that run between the toes, due to tight shoes and an inflamed or enlarged nerve. You may experience sharp knifelike or electrical-shock pain into the toes with walking that resolves when you take off your shoes. Or (less commonly) this condition can give you an achy, deep pain that radiates up to the back of your knee. Although sometimes a neuroma leads to surgery, home treatment is wider shoes and anti-inflammatories, such as Naproxen.

Bunion: A bunion is an enlargement of the soft tissue and bone around the joint between the toe and the foot bone (metatarsal). It is often associated with a deformity of the toe that drifts into a position crowding or overlying the second toe. Most bunions occur at the great toe junction, but lesser bunions can occur on the outside of the foot over the little toe junction. Pain is due to stretching of the soft tissues and to inflammation. So, again, the treatment is well-fitting, wide-toe-box shoes, and anti-inflammatories. Although foot doctors don't generally believe in them, I have found from personal experience that spacers placed between the great and second toes do help the pain. I never had a bunion in my life, having grown up mostly barefoot, and seldom wearing high-fashion, pointy-toed shoes. But at age fifty-five, when I became president of a national organization, I found myself wearing a suit and "pumps" frequently at meetings. After a weekend of meetings, I would have pain and swelling over my right great toe joint. I saw my friendly podiatrist, who agreed that it was a bunion. Not wanting surgery, I took an anti-inflammatory and put a spacer between my toes that took the stretching off the soft tissues that were inflamed. I avoided any dressy shoes for six weeks. At the end of that time, my pain was resolved.

There are two types of specialists who deal with foot and ankle problems—orthopaedic fellowship–trained foot and ankle surgeons, and podiatrists. Foot and ankle surgeons have one to two more years of surgical training after the five-year orthopaedic residency and four years of medical school. They are few and far between, often in university settings, and are fully involved in the government system. Podiatrists have four to five years of training and were traditionally cash based but, sadly, have begun to drink the Obamacare Kool-Aid. I think most podiatrists still do some cash practice and are more likely to be available in a meltdown. For the uncomplicated foot and ankle problems that you are most likely to develop, podiatrists generally do a very fine job and are much easier to access.

25

EAR INFECTIONS

One of my most memorable days as an intern was the day I cured "deafness." I was on call on ear, nose, and throat—properly known as *otorhinolaryngology* but generally called ENT. I was sitting in the on-call room with the third-year ENT resident when the phone rang. He answered, listened for a while, then asked, "What do the eardrums look like?" After hearing the caller's response, he said, "I think this sounds like an intern-to-intern problem; hold on," and he handed the phone to me. My fellow intern told me about a patient who had come to the ER complaining of sudden-onset deafness. He was fine the night before, but that morning suddenly could not hear. When I asked the intern the same question the resident had—"What do the eardrums look like?"—I realized why the phone was handed to me. My fellow intern (this wasn't perhaps his brightest moment) said to me in all seriousness, "I don't know. I can't see the eardrums because of all the wax." After looking disgustedly at the ENT resident, who was, by then, laughing pretty hard, I hung up, went to the ER, cleaned out the gentleman's ears, and voilà! He could hear again! The practice of medicine isn't always complicated; we just try to make it that way.

Earwax: Earwax is not a problem for everyone. The amount of wax production and the size and shape of the canal are genetically determined, so some people have more buildup than others. As in my internship story, one of the major problems is blockage of the external ear canal and thus blockage of sound hitting the tympanic membrane (eardrum). Q-tips, napkin corners, and other such things can actually push earwax deeper into the ear. But I still clean my wet ears with a soft Q-tip, and I doubt most people will give that up. So what do we do when we feel the ear canal is blocked with wax? Before I have a physician look in my ear, I mix equal parts of hydrogen peroxide and quite warm water. The resulting solution should be about body temperature—tepid but not hot to the touch. If you use cold water to irrigate the ear canal, you will induce severe vertigo (dizziness and room spinning). My fellow students and I did this for a test in medical school, and it was not pleasant—let me assure you. Use a blue bulb syringe and put the solution into the ear so you feel it bubbling. Let it sit for several minutes with you on your side, ear up. After that, use the rest of the solution to gently irrigate the canal, then tilt the ear down so any debris can drain into the sink or basin. If this doesn't work, you will need a physician. Do not use a bobby pin or any firm object in the ear canal. This can scratch the canal and lead to infection or perforate the eardrum.

Other foreign bodies in the ear are usually the result of children putting things such as dried beans in the ear. But occasionally insects will make their way into the outer ear canal. I keep a small surgical grasper called a *pituitary rongeur* for removing small things from small places. If the object is prominent, you can grab it with tweezers. *But do not scratch the ear canal wall in the attempt.* Small insects can be felt and heard by the victim, and they often can be flushed out with the same technique used for removing wax. In this case, you can just use warm water and tilt the ear to the sink. In inner cities the most common foreign body in the ear is a cockroach. Although through eons, the cockroach has adapted to all sorts of environmental challenges, it has never evolved enough to be able to back up. So if a cockroach crawls into your ear while you are sleeping, it has no way to go but inward. As an intern I became somewhat proficient at removing these with the pituitary rongeur—rather like fighting a fifteen-pound bass on a six-pound test line. If this happens to you with either a cockroach, a June bug (a more common scenario in the Midwest), or a similar bug, and you can reach it easily with tweezers, you can try getting it out. But remember: don't scratch the ear canal. If unsuccessful, you may have to seek medical attention for the proper tools and fishing skill.

Itching ears are usually due to dry skin. This often happens in the winter. If you are prone to eczema, itching ears may be a manifestation of sensitive allergy-prone skin. This is usually treated simply by swabbing the ear with a Q-tip dipped in a little 1 percent hydrocortisone (HC) cream. Don't do this frequently. Frequent use of steroid cream can thin the skin. I probably do this three to four days in a row once or twice a year at the most. It is also important not to let your ears stay moist. I know we are told not to put anything smaller than our elbows into our ears, but if people actually followed that advice, why are Q-tips still sold? Being curious, I did an informal poll of my medical colleagues and found that they *all* use Q-tips in their ears. So why do we persist in telling patients *not* to use Q-tips when we should be telling them *how* to use them? I dry my ears with Q-tips. I buy soft, good-quality ones, and I just don't try to push too deeply—just as far as the tip goes comfortably and without scratching the wall of the canal. If you are prone to trapping water in the ear after showering or swimming, use a swimmer's ear solution regularly. You can buy these in drugstores or make your own (see below).

To simplify the issue of ear infections, there are two general categories—external ear infections and internal ear infections. External ear infections involve the outer canal and can often be treated with topical medications. Internal ear infections are infections behind the eardrum and cannot be reached by topical treatment.

Internal ear infections are more complicated and generally require antibiotics. They will sometimes resolve on their own because some are viral. But if an untreated bacterial ear infection persists, it may perforate the eardrum and cause hearing loss—temporary or permanent. An internal ear infection may cause a sense of fluid or a "sloshing" sound in the ear. Some hearing loss is common. It may occur after a cold or allergy that causes the Eustacian tube (drainage tube from the ear) to be plugged. In this instance, fluid backs up into the middle ear and may bulge out the eardrum. This fluid then gets colonized with bacteria. Generally a Z-Pak (or a ten-day course of erythromycin, or penicillin if you are not allergic) will take care of the problem.

External ear infections: An external ear infection is in the outer canal, on the outside of the eardrum. Although it, too, can cause hearing loss when the canal is swollen, hearing loss is not the predominant feature. These infections just hurt. When you grasp the ear and wiggle it, it causes pain. You can sometimes see redness in the canal, but this is difficult without specialized equipment. These infections occur from bacteria getting into a canal that is moist for prolonged periods. Because swimmers often have water trapped in the canal, or at least the canal is wet from frequent exposure to water, external ear infections are common; hence, the name swimmer's ear. Although antibiotics are sometimes used in severe cases, the usual treatment is topical. Keep water out. Place Neosporin or bacitracin ointment on a Q-tip and carefully insert into the canal. If the canal is swollen, it may need a cloth wick—a short strip of fabric—with antibiotic ointment on it, pushed gently in farther and farther as the swelling recedes. A diluted vinegar solution—one part white vinegar to fifteen parts water to change the pH—can be used to soak the wick or flush the ear. If flushing the ear, use warm water to avoid giving yourself vertigo. If bad enough, use of antibiotics is warranted.

As a preventative measure, you can buy swimmer's ear solution in the pharmacy or make your own solution. This can also be used to dry up the infected canal once the very raw surface is calmed down.

HOMEMADE SWIMMER'S EAR SOLUTION
1/4 cup white vinegar
1/4 cup isopropyl alcohol
Combine in a small glass jar with a dropper lid. This will keep indefinitely. After swimming, put 3 to 4 drops in one ear. Let it rest for about 5 minutes, and then turn your head and repeat in the other ear.

It is important to take hearing issues seriously. It is said in medicine that more people commit suicide because of deafness than blindness. Blindness cuts you off from things, but deafness cuts you off from people. Hearing loss is generally caused by three things: genetics, noise exposure, or infection to the inner ear. You can't choose your parents, but you can choose to protect your hearing from loud noise. I have many ex-military friends who have hearing loss from exploding ordnance or jet noise. One of the common causes of hearing loss is loud music. Then there are saws and loud hair dryers and engine noise. Whenever possible, use ear protection. I know military pilots who wear both ear canal plugs and cranial ear protectors (appropriately called Mickey Mouse ears) over them. And finally, if your child has recurrent ear infections, don't just accept it. Have it evaluated. Sometimes drainage tubes prevent later hearing loss. Sometimes just a simple course of antibiotics is needed—but not always. When a child complains he can't hear, believe him. The consequence of being wrong can be a lifetime of isolation from conversation with others.

26

SORE THROATS

Most sore throats are viral, and no antibiotic will help. There is a tendency to treat all sore throats with antibiotics, but that is wrong and may make you allergic to an antibiotic you will need later in life.

In general, sore throats accompany colds. Rarely do they occur in isolation. The treatment is generally time, fluids, and a soothing solution or lozenge. Once again I caution you against using Tylenol for pain, given the new thinking about Tylenol's bad effect on the NMDA receptor in the brain. Instead, gargle with salt water. Simply add a teaspoon or two of salt to a warm glass of water and gargle. Topical sprays, such as Chloraseptic, can also help pain.

High doses of vitamin C can help. I can't prove this, but as noted in previous chapters, I bumped up my vitamin C dose and it helped me. The recommended daily allowance (RDA) for vitamin C is 65 milligrams a day—an intake level so low it does not saturate the white cells that fight off infection. The first thing white cells do in response to a problem is to suck in vitamin C from the surrounding environment. That's why I take more as a baseline, and I take at least 1,000 milligrams every hour or two when I am ill.

It also helps to get enough rest. Many young doctors know that they get sick as they get overworked—because their immune systems are not functioning optimally when the body is sleep deprived.

Some young people have very visible tonsils with pits, and these get filled with dead cells and debris and can become infected. This is one reason for removing tonsils. But tonsils are a line of defense for infection. When I was an overworked, sleep-deprived medical student, I had recurrent sore throats. I would look at my throat in the mirror with a flashlight and see enlarged tonsils that looked like sponges with white junk in the holes. I reasoned that the immune system cannot get into spaces without good blood supply (which is why we drain abscesses). I took a tongue depressor and systematically massaged the tonsils to remove the white debris as it accumulated, and over time my tonsils became invisible and my sore throats went away. I don't recommend this for everyone, but if you have this problem and can handle the tendency to gag, it does work.

For a sore throat that is persistent, has swelling, has any compromise of airway, or is accompanied by unrelenting fever, seek medical help.

27

ABSCESSES, BOILS, AND ZITS

An abscess is a pocket of pus that is walled off from the surrounding tissue. It can be acute or chronic, small or large, deep or superficial. Our bodies take care of small, superficial abscesses all the time, especially in the hand, when it expels a small splinter along with a little wisp of white pus. The most common abscesses we encounter in everyday life are due to a foreign body—like a splinter or a thorn—that penetrates the skin. When a small piece of wood or other material gets under the skin, the body sends white cells to attack this "invader." In the process these cells die and gel together, giving the characteristic yellowish-white pus. Often the pus pocket and surrounding inflammation are enough to cause the object to become loose under the skin and pushed to the surface. Sometimes, however, the abscess is beyond the body's capability to deal with. In this case the abscess will become bigger, painful, warm, and often soft in the center due to the pus. Sometimes infection will start to spread, and you will see redness streaking up the skin. *Boil* is a term generally used for abscesses that develop in the buttocks, usually around a clogged hair follicle.

Abscesses are benefited by the following, in order of progressively more aggressive treatment:

1. **Warmth** helps stimulate blood flow, which brings in more cells to fight the infection. Moisture helps soften the skin in case a track to the object can be opened. It also makes the skin more permeable for passage of the foreign body or for pus to drain. You can soak in a tub, put the extremity in a warm sink, apply a heating pad over a wrung-out wet washcloth, or simply apply a heating pad.

2. **Antibiotics:** In the age of antibiotics, the reason the world still needs surgeons like me is that *antibiotics do not penetrate into an abscess.* All they do is treat the surrounding area and help prevent the spread of infection, but they are only useful in small abscesses; the body itself must spit out the object, or the abscess must drain spontaneously through a small channel, and any antibiotics are used as an addition to (not in place of) the warm soaks.

3. **Surgical drainage** is needed for any abscess that is persistent, large, fluctuant (soft in the center, suggesting liquid pus), or accompanied by spreading redness. Usually this means seeking professional help. But sometimes, you may have a localized hot, red, swollen abscess with a very superficial pus pocket that can easily be unroofed and the pus released. Generations of farm wives have drained pus pockets in their kids and husbands by heating a hat pin on the stove to red-hot over a flame, cleansing the abscess, then pricking it with the sterile pin to cause the pus to come out. That technique still works. I have done that at home with my kids and myself. I use alcohol on the skin, but otherwise, all my surgical training doesn't add much to Grandma's hot pin idea. (I just happen to have 18-gauge surgical needles at home.) Don't get lazy with sterilization techniques. Use isopropyl alcohol on the skin and a sterile needle. Sterilize the needle by boiling it for ten minutes, heating it to red-hot, or swabbing it with isopropyl alcohol. Sometimes there is a very thin roof of dead skin over obvious pus. Make the biggest drainage hole you can make—piercing dead tissue doesn't hurt. Get rid of as much dead tissue as possible. Your patient will let you know when you get into

live skin! If you have a scalpel, this works better for bigger areas. Even surgeons do not usually use anesthetic in these cases because there are no nerve endings in dead skin, and anesthetic doesn't get into infected tissue well—plus, it hurts more to inject anesthetic than it does to do one quick jab to release the pus.

Once the pus is draining, sit in a tub (if the abscess is in the buttock, for example) to soak the area. Sometimes a 50 percent solution of hydrogen peroxide (equal parts water and hydrogen peroxide) can be used with a bulb syringe or standard hypodermic syringe to irrigate the wound. After draining a large abscess, pack the hole left behind with sterile gauze soaked in a mild soap solution (see sidebar) or in an acetic acid solution (see sidebar). Smaller abscesses are best treated with topical antibiotic gel. Any significant, spreading redness means *head for professional help*. If help is not available after doing all of the previous steps, start clindamycin (300 mg) three times a day and cipro (750 mg) twice a day.

MILD SOAP SOLUTION
3 to 4 drops mild antimicrobial soap (such as Hibiclens) or baby shampoo
1/2 cup water
Slowly stir the soap or shampoo into the water.

ACETIC ACID SOLUTION
1 ounce white vinegar
15 ounces water
Combine and use for treating abscesses and other abrasions.

"Zits" (or pimples) are actually a different kettle of fish. Acne and its variants cause swellings that look a lot like little abscesses, and maybe they are (I never quite learned that in medical school), but they are treated very differently. Generally, surgical drainage is not indicated. My son, in his senior year of medical school—with a little bit of knowledge but not quite enough—decided to do the hot pin trick to a progressively swelling facial lump. It looked for all the world like a deep abscess, but as he found out, poking at it made it worse. In general, isolated, firm facial swellings larger than the normal pimple need antibiotics (Keflex 500 mg four times a day, tetracycline 250 mg four times a day, or doxycycline 200 mg twice a day, or a combination of Cipro and Clindamycin as described above, until gone) and should not be squeezed, needled, stabbed, or in any way mechanically irritated. Topical treatment with metronidazole gel or clindamycin solution is helpful. Nothing, however, is more useful than a dermatologist or primary care provider who knows about skin and acne.

It is important to note that infections in the facial area drain into the venous system of the brain and can cause serious problems if bacteria seed the veins in the brain. If the infection seeds the cavernous sinus, a complex venous plexus at the base of the brain, it can cause a clot, from which one can die suddenly. As I entered puberty, my physician dad told me about this potential disastrous outcome to encourage me not to pinch pimples. So as other kids were worried about running with scissors, I was worried about dying suddenly of "cavernous sinus thrombosis."

In summary, don't "pop zits," be very attentive to unusual facial swelling, and in the medical meltdown don't hesitate to use your antibiotic store for anything that you think is a facial infection.

28

EMERGENCY DENTAL CARE

Dentistry is a highly specialized, technologically demanding field, so dental problems must always end up in "the chair." However, sometimes things happen at 2 a.m. on a Saturday, and you need a plan for the weekend.

Losing a tooth or a piece of a tooth spontaneously is usually not an emergency unless a tooth breaks in such way as to become painful. That generally means the *dentin*, or inside, of a vital (live) tooth has become exposed to the air. For a fractured and painful tooth, first rinse the area in warm water. (It may be very sensitive to cold.) There are over-the-counter waxy compounds that can be purchased at the pharmacy to temporarily cover the exposed dentin. In the absence of that, clove oil is a dental anesthetic. Soak a cotton ball in the oil of cloves and apply to the broken tooth. Ibuprofen (Motrin) is short acting but one of the best non-narcotic pain medicines.

Dental abscesses are one of the most painful of nature's plagues on humanity. My father was a physician and a research dentist who years ago helped develop the first fluoride toothpaste. (Unfortunately, although a professional student, he never attended law school and didn't understand patents well, so he lost out and I continue to work.) Ironically, I inherited my mother's strangely bad teeth that rot from within. I literally have had root canals for abscesses in every tooth in my head. I finally did the last five prophylactically because I got so tired of being in pain. And it solved the problem, but trust me when I tell you that *nothing* hurts like a bad tooth abscess—not even childbirth, and I've had both. Over the years I was on a first-name basis with endodontists all over the country, wherever I lived, and in the Navy. When I developed my last classic dental abscess, I woke up with some pain that got gradually worse in the morning. I called the endodontist for an appointment at 4 p.m. At 1 p.m., I showed up in the office, and when the secretary asked me why, I told her, "I have no place I can go like this. I'll just sit here, and maybe he can numb me up and let me wait. If not, I'll just sit without moving."

So, what to do? Well, first, is it the gum or the tooth? A piece of stuck popcorn or meat or some foreign particle jammed down into a gum may cause pain or a "periodontal" abscess that is all in the soft tissue—the teeth themselves being healthy. In my world of dental nightmares, I keep an oral irrigator machine in my bathroom that I use for routine periodontal (gum) care. (I like the Hydro Floss super-duty pulse lavage machine.) Most people who lose their teeth later in life do so, not because the teeth rot, but because the gums have chronic disease, recede, and expose the roots of the teeth and cause teeth loosening. I cannot recommend an oral irrigator enough. For an acute problem I recommend doing warm water pulse lavages with a small amount of hydrogen peroxide in the water, and thoroughly rinsing (lavaging) around the offending area. Then do some self-diagnostics. First, push on the gum around the area. Then tap on the teeth one at a time and see if you can find one that causes pain. Try some ice water in the area—does that make it worse? In short, if only the gum causes pain, it may be local inflammation. If ice makes it worse and/or tapping on the tooth hurts (warning: that may send you through the roof), it's most likely a tooth abscess. A tooth that is cracked into the root may also be the cause, but this tends to become painful and level off. The bad thing about a tooth abscess is that once it gets started, it produces "pus under pressure" in an area with a ton of nerve endings. "Pain" is such an insufficient word. I asked one dentist to just cut my head off because it hurt so badly. The good news is, with drainage and appropriate dental care, pain is generally relieved right away.

If you have an abscess, you will have to get to a dentist. For pain, try ibuprofen (800 mg) four times a day. This does two things—it relieves the pain, and it helps reduce the inflammation around the tooth. If you have a narcotic at home and need to temporize till Monday or the next morning, you have my sympathy. Take it as recommended and realize you cannot drive or put yourself into any dangerous situations—like climbing on the roof or signing divorce decrees. Lie still. Pain is worsened by activity. It may help to sleep sitting up a bit. If all of that fails and you don't have an emergency dentist to consult, go to the emergency room.

A permanent tooth that has been knocked out is an emergency because often the tooth can be replaced. Current recommendations are to pick the tooth up by the crown, avoiding touching the root. If you can rinse it and put it back into the socket, do so. If you cannot, it is best to drop the tooth into a small container of milk or, as a last resort, wrap the tooth in a moist cloth, taking care to protect the delicate soft tissues attached to the root. Call for an emergency dentist.

A bitten tongue is generally not an emergency unless you cannot stop the bleeding. Pressure for three minutes is the magic treatment. Then just give it time to heal and avoid reinjury.

Preventative dental care is the best way to avoid these issues. I have "dental religion" after a bunch of root canals and four implants that replace three teeth lost to abscess. My routine is nightly brushing with a non-fluoride toothpaste. (My dad's research aside, I believe fluoride is a carcinogen. He didn't have the statistics on inorganic fluoride in 1945.[1]) I floss daily, and for flossing after meals, I carry Doctor's Brush Picks, which work better around my implants. At night I usually use the Hydro Floss with tepid water. While driving, I use whitening trays that are lined with a hydrogen peroxide gel. Typically, you wear a whitening tray for twenty minutes a day. These are not cheap, but neither are the consequences of periodontal disease. Finally, I get my teeth professionally cleaned and checked twice a year. Even if you do it only yearly, it is better than nothing, and it may be adequate if you are compulsive about your gum care and do not accumulate much plaque buildup on your teeth. I don't chew gum routinely, but when I do, I chew only a xylitol gum that actually decreases bacteria in the mouth. I also try to avoid sweets and simple carbs.

Fortunately, many dentists are still amenable to cash payment, and insurance doesn't cover everything. But as dental insurance becomes more common and the government pays for more dental care (they do now for indigent children), we will face a dental melt-down, with shortages of dentists and restriction of care. Dentists are already facing the draconian actions of the federal government. Several years ago, the Association of American Physicians and Surgeons—a group that counts Ron Paul and Rand Paul as members and me as a past president—helped free a dentist from jail who had been in nearly solitary confinement *for five years*. He had been charged with "Medicaid fraud," but at the time of his release, the government could only prove he had overcharged Medicaid around thirty-five dollars. So dentists, welcome to the new world order in which physicians have lived for decades.

29

THE FUTURE OF MEDICINE

Where do we go from here? I doubt we can return to a true free market in medicine without literally a regime change. Sadly, as Russians and Chinese are in the process of privatizing their medical care, we are sliding down into the rat hole of medical socialism. As more physicians and surgeons opt out of seeing patients on government-paid plans, the politicians will get more complaints from constituents unable to access care. And they will take draconian steps. I doubt our politician over-lords will suddenly have a Zen moment of enlightenment and decide to institute free-market reforms. No, sadly, I think they will come down hard on the states—demanding that state medical boards not license physicians unless they take Medicare, Medicaid, Obamacare, Tricare, and any other government program that comes along.

There will be a wave of retirements—myself included—and partial retirements or slowdowns among those a little younger. Following that, we will have a new generation of physicians raised on electronic medical records, inefficiency, shoddy quality of care, and a nine-to-five mentality. These newly minted docs will not remember the great tenets of Osler, and they will take a modern, watered-down Hippocratic oath that fits today's socialist medical narrative. Sadly I am watching as my son completes medical school, and I see how little practical training he is receiving—compared to my education in the mid 1970s and 1980s. Had he not come to my hospital for some hands-on skills, he would not have learned to insert an IV catheter. His professors spend more time wrestling with the electronic medical records system than teaching him. He has been told that he should plan on another year of specialty training after a five-year general surgery residency so he will have enough experience to safely practice.

Remember when Obama and Nancy Pelosi said the new health care law would lower prices, improve quality, and increase "access"? What a joke. It is not doing any of these things. It is the last nail in the coffin of our freedom. If you owe your very health to the government, what else is there? At every level of medical care, we are being dumbed down by regulations that keep us from being efficient and effective. The stress put on physicians is causing record suicides and retirements. We are about to fall.

As T. S. Eliot wrote:

This is the way the world ends
This is the way the world ends
This is the way the world ends
Not with a bang but with a whimper.[1]

The whimper is from a patient lying in the hallway in an over-crowded hospital, or a baby in distress, born far from any obstetrician or pediatrician. The whimper is also from the physician who once treated patients the old-fashioned way—with concern, compassion, and competence—in an analog world of individuals, and his psyche cannot take the paradigm shift into Obamacare's digital medical system that sees patients as faceless ciphers.

What is about to happen is the result, not of too little government, but of too much. You and I have to be prepared. As the genius of practical living, Ben Franklin said, "By failing to prepare, you are preparing to fail." People tend to think of history following a gentle sine wave, varying little from day to day. Psychologically we expect tomorrow to be pretty much like today. But a quick look at the world shows a very different picture. Nearly overnight Sarajevo went from being a modern city to a bombed-out shell. Brits sipped gin and tonics and ate crumpets, ignoring Winston Churchill's warnings against downsizing their army, and overnight they were caught with their proverbial pants down as the world changed with Hitler's march into Poland. In 1860, America was prospering and developing like no nation on earth, and in the course of a few months was convulsed by a bloody civil war. Flappers danced and tycoons strutted right up until Black Friday and the stock market collapse. Members of the Russian aristocracy were suddenly made serfs to the Bolsheviks. My friend from Cambodia was the daughter of a well-to-do government official until the Khmer Rouge took him, and she was smuggled out of a nation that had devolved into the "killing fields." In short, if plotted on a graph, the world is not a sine wave but a "fractal landscape," with sudden, unexpected drop-offs.

I grew up with parents who lived through the Depression. It has always been my habit to be frugal, to conserve, to eat what's on my plate, and to be prepared for the unexpected financial catastrophe. But now I realize we must be prepared for the medical catastrophe that is of our own government's making.

I hope to see a future with freedom restored. Win, lose, or draw, I will no longer vote for people who enslave my children and unborn grandchildren to taxes and regulation and forced government-run health care. I plan to be as independent of the collapsing system as possible and to be able to offer my medical services to my neighbors, my friends, and my family, as well as for barter. I pray for God's blessing on our nation in this troubled time, and I hope this book will facilitate your well-being and even survival in the coming medical meltdown.

APPENDIX A

FURTHER READING AND OTHER RESOURCES

Maltsev, Yuri N. "What Soviet Medicine Teaches Us." *Mises Daily,* June 22, 2012, http://mises.org/daily/3650/What-Soviet-Medicine-Teaches-Us.

Maltsev, Yuri N. "Lessons from Soviet Medicine," *Journal of American Physicians and Surgeons*, 16, no. 2, (2011), http://www.jpands.org/vol16no2/maltsev.pdf.

Hieb, Lee D., MD. "Government Medicine is Hazardous to Your Health." *AAPS Online,* December 22, 2011, http://www.aapsonline.org/index.php/site/article/government_medicine_is_hazardous_to_your_health/.

Hieb, Lee D., MD. "Access to Care: the 3 Cs." *Journal of American Physicians and Surgeons,* 17, no. 3 (2012): 80-81. http://www.jpands.org/vol17no3/hieb.pdf.

Orient, Jane. "Obamacare: What is in It?" *Journal of American Physicians and Surgeons,* 15, no. 3 (2010): 87-93. http://www.jpands.org/vol15no3/orient.pdf.

Weber, Ralph. *Medicrats: Medical Bureaucrats that Rule Your Health Care*, ed. Dave Racer (Saint Paul, MN: Alethos Press, 2011).

Hieb, Lee D., MD. "Letter To Hospital Authorities on Mandatory Flu Vaccination." *Journal of American Physicians and Surgeons,* 18, no. 2 (2013): 47-49. http://www.jpands.org/vol18no2/hieb.pdf.

Hieb, Lee D., MD. *Tales from the Surgeon's Lounge and Collected Writings,* (Tuckahoe, NY: RJ Communications, 2013).

ANTI-AGING REFERENCES
Hieb, Lee D. MD. "Feds Keeping People Sick: The Vitamin D Story." *WND,* December 12, 2012. http://www.wnd.com/2012/12/feds-keeping-people-sick-the-vitamin-d-story/. Once you go to this site you can access the Archives for my older articles. There are many on anti-aging subjects.

Davis, William, MD. *Wheat Belly: Lose the Wheat, Lose the Weight, and Find Your Way Back to Health.* (Emmaus, PA: Rodale Books, 2014).

Perlmutter, David, MD. *Grain Brain: The Surprising Truth about Wheat, Carbs, and Sugar – Your Brain's Silent Killers.* (New York, NY: Little, Brown and Company, 2013).

Eades, Michael R., MD and Mary Dan Eades, MD. *Protein Power: The High Protein/Low Carbohydrate Way to Lose Weight, Feel Fit, and Boost Your Health – in Just Weeks!* (New York, NY: Bantam Books, 1997).

WorldHealth.net is the site for the American Academy of Anti-Aging Medicine. A4M is a nonprofit organization dedicated to the advancement of technology to detect, prevent, and treat aging-related disease. They have a library of information and a list of doctors you can access.

Cenegenics (Cenegenics.com) pioneered the development of Age Management Medicine (AMM) and has anti-aging medical clinics around the country.

OTHER RESOURCES
Poison Control Center
1-800-222-1222

SUPPLEMENTS

Life Extension Foundation (www.LEF.org) is a great source for information and for good quality supplements at a reasonable price. If you use my initials LDH as code, you can get a six-month free membership. They have a wonderful journal that teaches you the latest about anti-aging lifestyle.

Good Health Supplements (www.goodhealthsupplements.com) is a trusted source for good nutritional supplements that will help you maintain your health. They offer affordable, leading-edge technology in healthy heart support, breakthrough anti-aging, superior multivitamin, invaluable digestive supplementation and more, including Parent Essential Oils (PEOs). PEOs are probably a better alternative to fish oil.

CASH DOCTORS RESOURCES

The Association of American Physicians and Surgeons (www.AAPSonline.org) is a nonpartisan professional association of physicians in all types of practices and specialties across the country. It is the site for the free-market medicine doctors. They are developing a list of cash physicians in various areas of the country.

The DocCost (www.DocCost.com) concept was born in 2008 as a potential free-market solution to the ever-rising cost of health care in the United States. They help patients who are willing to pay cash at the time of service find doctors and other heath care providers that allow patients to compare charges.

MediBid (www.MediBid.com) gives health savings account and self-pay patients access to doctors who will provide them with quality medical care and upfront, cash pricing. It allows you to bid for surgical services and other procedures such as a colonoscopy with cash-only surgeons and physicians. www.MediBid.com

SOURCES FOR MANUALS AND EQUIPMENT

Special Operations Forces Medical Handbook

The Special Operations Forces Medical Handbook, 2001, is the first edition of a comprehensive medical reference resource designed for Special Operations Forces (SOF) medics. This "single-source" reference provides many revolutionary approaches to accessing medical information, such as a treatment hierarchy based on available medical resources and mission circumstances commonly facing the SOF medic and victims of the medical meltdown.

Available to download at http://www.nh-tems.com/documents/Manuals/SOF_Medical_Handbook.pdf

US Army First Aid Manual

The U.S. Army First Aid Manual offers skills and knowledge necessary for many life-threatening situations, with an emphasis on treating oneself and aiding others. Of use to soldiers in the field, to outdoorsmen, or to anyone in a dangerous situation without a medical professional on hand. This is the official manual for treating every type of injury and affliction in the field.

Available to download at http://1oro1.com/images/pdf%20files/FM%2021-11.pdf

Facemasks and N95 respirators are devices that may help prevent the spread of viruses and bacteria from one person to another. They are one part of an infection-control strategy that should also include frequent hand washing and social distancing.

You can find these masks online at N-95 Masks: http://www.fullsource.com/disposable-n95-masks/kimberly-clark-62126kc2/

The Grossnan Sinus Irrigator

The Grossnan Hydro Pulse Sinus System is the first pulsating system specifically for nasal and sinus irrigation. Not just a cleanse or rinse, the pulsating action is clinically proven to make your sinus cilia—the body's first line of defense against contagions, pollen, and foreign matter—work better. You can purchase this product on Amazon or at www.hydromedonline.com.

The Hydro Floss

Hydromagnetic oral irrigation treats the water magnetically, which affects the ionization process, which, in turn, reduces surface tension and inhibits the ability of the bacteria to bond and colonize and the calculus to form. You can purchase this product on Amazon or at www.hydrofloss.com.

SAM Splint

The SAM (Structural Aluminum Malleable) Splint is a compact, lightweight, highly versatile device designed for immobilizing bone and soft tissue injuries in emergency settings. You can purchase this product on Amazon or at www.sammedical.com.

Israeli Battle Bandage Dressing

The Israeli Bandage is an innovative, combat-proven first aid device for the staunching of blood flow from traumatic hemorrhage wounds in prehospital emergency situations. You can purchase this product on Amazon or at http://www.chinookmed.com or http://www.israelifirstaid.com.

Water BOB Fresh Water storage system

The waterBOB is a water containment system that holds up to 100 gallons of fresh drinking water in virtually any bathtub in the event of an emergency. You can purchase this product on Amazon or at www.waterbob.com.

Water Treatment Tablets

Potable Aqua iodine water disinfection tablets were developed by Harvard University in conjunction with the US Army in the 1940s, and have been used by the military for emergency drinking water disinfection for more than fifty years. You can purchase this product on Amazon or at www.potableaqua.com.

Radiation Dosimeter "RadSticker"

The RADStickerTM peel & stick, instant color-developing dosimeter, is always ready and with you 24/7, stuck onto the back of your driver's license or anything you keep close, for any future radiation emergency. You can purchase this product on Amazon or at http://disasterpreparer.com/radsticker/.

APPENDIX B

EMERGENCY KITS AND SUPPLEMENTS

STANDARD 72-HOUR SUPPLY KIT (NONMEDICAL)

Batteries

Candles

Drinking water

Emergency radio

Emergency rations such as 2,400-calorie food bars

First aid kit (if not using a separate medical kit, see page 247)

Moist towelettes in resealable container or individually wrapped

Antiseptic wipes

Pocket tissue

Pocketknife

Waterproof matches

Rope

Dust masks

Duct tape

Clothespins

Flashlight

Gloves

Poncho

Survival blankets

Tube tent

Water purification tablets

Whistle

MEDICAL 72-HOUR SUPPLY KIT

ACE wrap (three 4-inch wraps)

Afrin nasal spray

Aleve or Naproxen 500 mg

Antibiotic ointment

Band-Aids

Cetirizine

Chewable vitamin C (500 mg)

Chlotrimazole 1% antifungal cream

Cipro 500 or 750 mg tabs

Clindamycin 300 mg tabs

Gauze bandages (1 dozen, 4 x 4 inches)

Hydrocortisone Cream

Iodine supplement 12.5 mg

Melatonin 3 mg sublingual

N-95 masks

Prescription medicines (in daily-dose zip lock snack bags—enough for at least two to three weeks)

Q-tips

SAM Splint (4 x 36 inches)

Sling

Special Operations Forces Medical Handbook (see page 241) or *US Army First Aid Manual* (see page 242)

Vitamin D$_3$ (5,000 IU for children and 10,000 IU for adults)

Water purification tablets

AUTHORIZED MEDICAL ALLOWANCE LISTS (AMALS)

Prescription Drugs

If you take a lot of prescription drugs or hormones, make an AMAL just for daily drugs, and put all the rest in another AMAL for drugs used only in unusual situations. That way you can rotate easily old drugs for new. Put EpiPens on top and rotate by expiration date.

PERSONAL

Personal hormones

Personal prescriptions: (for example, thyroid, blood pressure, and/or glaucoma medication, anticoagulants, eye drops)

ANTIBIOTICS

Amoxicillin 500 mg tablet

Cipro 500 or 750 mg tablets

Clindamycin 300 mg tablets

Doxycycline 100 mg tablets

PAIN AND SWELLING

Codeine (save extras from procedures and keep in secure place)

Ibuprofen 400 mg or Naproxen 500 mg (which is better for anti-inflammatory and swelling but not as immediate relief of pain.)

Migraine medications

SEVERE RESPIRATORY ALLERGIES

EpiPen

OVER-THE-COUNTER (OTC) DRUGS

Cough and cold

Afrin nasal spray

Children's nasal spray

Liquid cough and cold medicine that does not contain Tylenol

Throat lozenges

GASTROINTESTINAL

Mylanta (immediate-relief antacid)

Omeprazole (stomach acid)

Senekot-S (for constipation)

ANTI-INFLAMMATORY

Baby aspirin 81 mg

Naproxen or Aleve 220 mg

ALLERGY

Benadryl 25 mg tablets (drowsy)

Cetirizine (nondrowsy)

SLEEP/STRESS

Melatonin 3 mg sublingual tablets (to get to sleep)

5-HTP, 50 to 100 mg (to stay asleep, and for stress; can be taken in the day)

L-theonine (for brain calming and sleep, see LEF.org)

OINTMENTS, SKIN PRODUCTS, AND WOUND CARE

Pharmacy items

ACE wrap (3-inch and 4-inch)

Adhesive strips (like Steri-Strips, 1/2-inch and 1/4-inch for closing wounds)

Antibiotic ointment (Neosporin, bacitracin, polymixin, or polysporin)

Antifungal (miconazole nitrate 2%)

Band-Aids

Calamine lotion (for bug bites and poison ivy)

Chlorhexidine 0.12% oral rinse (can be purchased OTC for pets)

Clean cloths

Cling gauze

Ear bulb syringe

Gauze sponges (2-inch square and 4-inch square)

Gauze sponges with petroleum to prevent sticking (1 x 8-inch Xeroform gauze)

Hydrocortisone cream 1%

Hydrogen peroxide

Isopropyl alcohol

Israeli Battle Bandage Dressing (optional for major wounds)

Micropore tape (1-inch wide, used for bandages)

Q-tips

Skin cream or lotion (unscented)

Scissors

Silver Solution kit, optional (see appendix C)

Syringes (half-dozen 10 ml with 18-gauge needles)

Metal sterilizable basin or small metal bowl

HOUSEHOLD ITEMS
Aloe vera plant (for superficial burns)
Baking soda
Honey (to be used as an antibiotic for infected wounds)
Mustard (for burns)
Salt
Xylitol crystals (at least 1 pound)
Vaseline

SPLINTS
Aircast ankle brace
Arm sling
ACE wraps (4-inch)
CAM Boot
SAM Splint (4 x 36 inches)

DISINFECTANTS AND WATER PURIFICATION
Bleach (for disinfecting surfaces, containers, or drinking water, see sidebar)
White vinegar (for disinfecting use a 1:8 ratio or 2 cups per gallon of water)
WaterBOB fresh water storage system (see page 243)
Water treatment tablets (iodine tablets to treat water)

CLOROX SOLUTION
For disinfecting doorknobs, toys, countertops etc.: Add 1/2 cup of bleach per gallon of water or 1½ teaspoons per cup of water.
For drinking water: After letting the water settle so there is no particulate matter floating, add 2 drops bleach per quart (4 cups) or water or 8 drops bleach per gallon of water.

INFORMATION AND TESTING EQUIPMENT
The American Medical Association Handbook of First Aid and Emergency Care
American College of Physicians Complete Home Medical Guide
Special Operations Forces Medical Handbook

US Army First Aid Manual
Nonbattery thermometers
Radiation dosimeter cards
Measuring tape
Stethoscope, blood pressure cuff, depending on level of expertise

REPIRATORY CARE
Inhalers (prescription)
Nebulizer with Albuterol (or other prescribed bronchodilator)
Oxygen generator (if dependent on an oxygen tank)

PET CARE (OPTIONAL)
Pet prescription medicines
Ear mite solution
Worming medication

SUPPLEMENTS EVERYONE SHOULD TAKE
These recommendations are intended for healthy people over age five. I don't usually recommend multivitamins, but prefer specific supplements. However, if food is scarce and you are eating a survival-type diet, it would be good to take a good multivitamin daily to supplement trace elements. I don't recommend giving supplements to children under the age of three. For children over three years of age, a children's multivitamin without iron is a good idea especially if there is a less-than-optimal diet. Also there is lots of evidence to recommend fish oil for children. I like Nortdic Natural's supplement that includes fish oil (EPA, DHA, GLA) as well as vitamin D_3 1,000 IU. You can buy this in health food stores or order online at omega-direct.net/prod_completed3jr.html. If you have a significant chronic disease or renal failure, or for children under the age of three, consult your physician.

VITAMIN	DAILY DOSE
VITAMIN C	1000 MG (ADULTS)
VITAMIN C	500 MG (CHILDREN AGES 8 AND UP)
IODINE IN THE FORM OF IODORAL	12.5MG
VITAMIN D3	10,000 IU (ADULTS)
VITAMIN D3	5000 IU (CHILDREN AGES 8 AND UP)
ZINC	7–15 MG
FISH OIL OR PREFERABLY PEOS	3000 MG (ADULT) (DOSE DEPENDENT ON PARTICULAR FORMULATION)
FISH OIL	3000 MG (CHILDREN)
SUBLINGUAL B12 (USUALLY MIXED WITH FOLATE AND SELENIUM)	1,000 MG (ADULTS OVER 50 YEARS OF AGE)
LYSINE	1000 MG
B COMPLEX	RECOMMENDED DOSE

OPTIONAL SUPPLEMENTS

I take more than the above supplements because I choose to spend my disposable income on my health and longevity. The above short list I would pay for no matter what. But these are optional unless you have been diagnosed with specific deficiencies.

VITAMIN	DAILY DOSE	BENEFIT
CDP CHOLINE	250 MG	BRAIN HEALTH
R ALPHA LIPOIC ACID	250 MG	FREE RADICAL SCAVENGER TO DECREASE AGING
CO-Q10	100 MG	SUPPORTS MITOCHONDRIAL METABOLISM
CURCUMEN (OR 1 TBSP TURMERIC HEATED IN A LITTLE OLIVE OIL AND BLACK PEPPER	800 TO 1,000 MG	AN ALL PURPOSE ANTI-AGING SUPPLEMENT ANTI-OXIDANT AND FREE RADICAL SCAVENGER— MUCH ADVISED BY DR. BLAYLOCK IN HIS ANTI-AGING NEWSLETTER FOR A VARIETY OF ISSUES
FLUSH FREE NIACIN	500 MG	FOR OPTIMIZING LIPIDS, ENERGY PRODUCTION AND DNA REPAIR
GAMMA E	400 MG	THE CORRECT ANTI-OXIDANT FORM OF VITAMIN E
MAGNESIUM CITRATE	800 MG	ELDERLY PEOPLE SEEM TO BE DEFICIENT IN MAGNESIUM AND I SUSPECT IT IS DIETARY. IT IS MAJOR PLAYER IN PREVENTING HYPERTENSION
N-ACETYL CYSTEINE	600 MG	SUPPLIES SUBSTRATE TO MAKE A MAJOR BRAIN ANTI-OXIDANT— GLUTATHIONE
PHOSPHATIDYL SERINE	150 MG	SUPPORTS BRAIN HEALTH
RESVERATROL	200 MG	LONGEVITY
SAM-E	400 MG	BRAIN HEALTH
TAURINE	1,000 MG	ESSENTIAL AMINO ACID, HIGH CONCENTRATION IN THE EYE
EPICORE	500 MG	AN IMMUNE ENHANCER/OPTIMIZER

APPENDIX C

RECIPES AND FORMULAS

1/4 PERCENT ACETIC ACID SOLUTION

An acetic acid solution is a mild antibacterial that helps keep infections at bay and kills harmful bacteria.

1 ounce white vinegar

15 ounces clean water

Add the vinegar to the water and mix well. Store in a clean jar with a tight-fitting lid. This will keep indefinitely.

COLLOIDAL SILVER SOLUTION

Colloidal silver is a suspension of submicroscopic metallic silver particles in a colloidal base. The silver helps thwart fungus in the body and is considered by some to be a powerful antibacterial and antiviral solution. I don't take it internally, but use it for wounds and dressings. It can be a very effective sinus disinfectant as an alternative to the Sinus Irrigation Solution (see page 254), *but* do not use it for more than a few days, because silver, when absorbed, causes Algerolism (formerly known as Argerolism from the name of the silver-containing nasal drops) a permanent generalized blue deposition of silver in the skin. You do not want this. I have seen people with it, and they look vaguely Smurf-like. You can get kits to make this solution, but I prefer this simple setup:

1 quart mason jar

2 large-gauge pure (not sterling) silver wires

2 alligator clips

3 to 4 9-volt batteries

9-volt battery connector

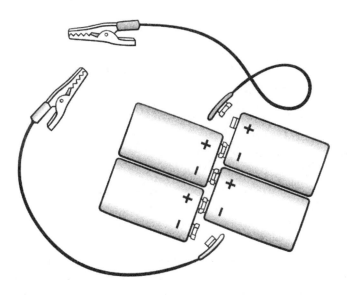

1. As in the above picture, the batteries are clamped together in series using the attachments on the batteries—positive to negative to positive to negative so you have left over one positive and one negative.

2. At one end connect an alligator clamp to a red wire, and at the other an alligator clamp to a black wire.

3. Fill the mason jar three-quarters full with *distilled* water.

4. Suspend the silver wires over the lip of the jar on either side; the bottom 4 inches of the wires should be submerged in the solution. Attach an alligator clamp to each wire and allow it to sit overnight.

5. In the morning you should have a faintly brown solution that you can use for soaking dressing or to use for sinus irrigation. I know people who have dramatically improved arthritis and chronic sinus infection from drinking 2 to 3 ounces of colloidal silver daily for four to five days, but I would be leery of doing this for fear of toxicity from silver deposition. I use it topically.

SINUS IRRIGATION SOLUTION

This is a good solution that can be used to clear out your sinuses. It can be made in bulk and stored in an airtight plastic container. If you have chronic sinusitis you probably should do a flush twice daily until clear. If you just have seasonal issues, do it daily during the season to keep the turbinates (the lumpy lining of the nasal passages) free of pollen and other allergens, and to keep the sinuses unblocked. If you have chronic sinus problems a Grossnan Sinus Pulse Irrigator is well worth the expense. I cured my long-standing sinus issue this way. Or, if your problem is very mild, you could use a NetiPot or sinus rinse kit found at any drug store. The salt and soda combination in this solution is gentle on the tissues, and the xylitol is a non-nutrient substance that is taken up by bacteria but gives them no real energy to reproduce.

1/3 cup salt
1/3 cup baking soda
1/3 cup xylitol crystals

Combine the ingredients and store in a sealable plastic bag or other airtight container. To use, mix 1 to 1½ teaspoons of the mixture into 16 ounces of warm water and follow the directions on your irrigator or NetiPot.

Note: If you are having an active infection, e.g., blowing out yellow or greenish thick mucus and having pain and fever, it helps to add a few drops of chlorhexidine 0.12% to the solution. (This is by prescription used primarily for periodontal disease, but the bacteria that infect sinuses are often the same, or at least respond to this. Most physicians should not have a problem if you ask for a prescription for it. However, the same strength chlorhexidine rinse can be purchased over the counter for pet dental rinse. An 8-ounce bottle is roughly $20 and should last a long time, depending on the frequency of use.)

MY EASY-PEASY SOAP RECIPE

Makes about a year's supply of soap for two people

For the soap molds, I just use glass baking dishes or cardboard boxes lined with waxed paper. But if you want nicer looking soap, you can use store-bought molds or make molds. I've seen someone use a section of a rain gutter stood on end for a mold. The number of bars is variable depending on the size you choose, and each bar lasts two or three times as long as store-bought soap. In my household, now with just two of us, this batch of soap lasted a year.

The first thing to be aware of is that lye is very caustic. It will burn skin upon contact. Always use gloves and eye protection. Never add water to lye. Always add lye to water, and do so in a well-ventilated area (outside is preferable).

1 pound lye crystals
2 pints water
5 3/4 pounds lard
2 1/2 cups pure olive oil
cooking thermometer
soap molds

Pour the lye crystals into the water while stirring constantly. Because the lye water solution produces an exothermic chemical reaction, the solution becomes warm to hot. This solution needs to cool to about 85 degrees.

While the lye water is cooling, start melting the lard in another pot until it is at 90 degrees. (I use my grandmother's old blue-speckled canning pot.)

The point is to have the lard and the lye solution at about the same temperature. Some people do this at a higher temperature of 130 degrees.

Slowly pour the lye solution into the lard while mixing. I use a stick blender that I bought just for this purpose and leave it in the pot when not in use. But before this I used my kitchen hand mixer and cleaned it afterward. (You are making soap after all.) This mixing may take 30 minutes or more.

When the mixture is smooth and creamy and thick, pour it into the molds. I don't add color or fragrance because I want pure hypoallergenic soap.

Put the molds in an out-of-the-way place (I use my spare bathtub) and cover with a wool blanket. That increases the temperature and speed of the process of saponification (becoming soap), which will occur mostly during the first 3 days. If the soap is hard at that point, remove and cut into the size pieces you want. Then put them in a cardboard box in layers separated by wax paper or brown paper. Let them sit for 4 weeks before using. Saponification happens slowly over these weeks, but once completed, the soap will last for many months and will be a great-feeling smooth hard soap.

SWIMMER'S EAR SOLUTION
1/4 cup white vinegar
1/4 cup isopropyl alcohol

Combine in a small glass jar with a dropper lid. This will keep indefinitely. After swimming, put 3 to 4 drops in one ear. Let it rest for about 5 minutes, and then turn your head and repeat in the other ear.

OUR FAVORITE GLUTEN-FREE BREAD

This recipe is courtesy of Domata Flour. There are other recipes for gluten-free breads at www.domataglutenfree.com/recipes.html. All the ingredients should be brought to room temperature.

3 cups sifted Domata Recipe Ready Flour
1/2 cup nonfat dry milk powder
3/4 teaspoon salt
1 1/2 teaspoons baking powder
3/4 teaspoon unflavored gelatin
2 tablespoons sugar
3 eggs, beaten
3/4 teaspoon vinegar
1/8 cup vegetable oil
1 1/4 cups plus 1/8 cup lukewarm water
3 1/2 teaspoons Saf instant yeast

Grease a 5 x 9-inch loaf pan, and dust with flour.

Combine the flour, dry milk, salt, baking powder, gelatin, and sugar in your mixing bowl and let it sit for several minutes while preparing the wet ingredients. Whisk together the eggs, vinegar, oil, and water. Add the yeast; then add them to the dry mixture and stir for *only* 1 minute. *Do not overmix.* The batter should be slightly thicker than the consistency of cake batter.

If necessary, add water a tablespoon at a time, as needed, to achieve this texture. Spoon the batter into the prepared pan, smooth with wet fingers, cover, and let rise in a warm place until the dough reaches the top of the pan, about 60 minutes.

Preheat oven to 400 degrees. Bake for 10 minutes; then cover lightly with foil and bake for another 35 to 40 minutes, depending on your oven. Remove from pan immediately to cool before slicing. Store tightly covered on the counter for 3 days, in freezer for several weeks. (It will dry out in the refrigerator).

MAKING YOUR OWN GLUTEN-FREE FLOUR

I love Domata gluten-free flour, and I definitely recommend it for beginning to cook gluten-free. But to save some money I often make my own gluten-free flour. Here is my general formula:

35% white rice flour (2 1/4 cups)
30% brown rice flour (1 3/4 cups)
30% tapioca flour (1 3/4 cups)
3% guar gum or xanthan gum or a combination of the two (3 tablespoons)
2% pectin (2 tablespoons)

Sometimes I add some cornstarch as well. Although I attached numbers to give you a feel for proportions, honestly I've gotten to the point that I simply add to my bin as it gets low, and don't do too much measuring. This is not rocket science. I suppose the purists will get better bread results by getting the perfect mix, but I'm not that picky. I get rice flour pretty cheaply at the local Asian market. Guar gum and xanthan gum can be purchased at large specialty groceries but I get mine on line. Pectin is used in canning and is generally locally available. You can also add some nut flours for different tastes and recipes. Nut flours add fat to the mix so shouldn't be used in things like piecrust or French bread. I tried potato starch once and hated the taste, so I never use that. I added sorghum flour once and didn't think the bread was as light and fluffy, but you can experiment. In any case by making your own you do save a lot of money. I still use Domata when cooking for guests or gifting and a perfect first-time outcome is required.

DR. PERLMUTTER'S COCONUT MILK MOUSSE

1 (15-ounce) can full-fat coconut milk
3 tablespoons cocoa powder
1 to 2 teaspoons stevia

Chill the can of coconut milk overnight. Scoop out the thickened milk and whip with mixer till smooth and a mousse-like consistency.

Add three tablespoons of cocoa powder and the stevia to taste. Whip again and chill in small ramekins.

He has other recipes in his book *Grain Brain* that is well worth reading to preserve your brain health and more.

APPENDIX D

A SAMPLE MEDICAL RECORD YOU MAKE FOR YOURSELF

Today's medical world is being held captive to electronic medical records thanks to Obamacare and other federal government programs that mandate conversion to digital records. I recently had a physical, and after years of going to the same provider, this time they had no record of my medications and allergies because they had implemented the mandatory electronic medical record. Because these electronic records are notoriously inaccurate, unavailable, or indecipherable, for your safety I recommend a single-page well-organized medical record that you can keep in your wallet or purse and take to all your doctor visits. (If you have many health issues, it may be longer. But keep it to two pages at the very most. More than that, and a busy emergency room doctor's eyes will glaze over.) The point of this record is to provide a useful concise summary, not a life history of everything you have had happen to you medically. Brevity is the soul of both wit and a good medical review.

When you list medications, do not list all your vitamins or supplements. You can tell that to someone when and if you are admitted to the hospital, but it is not a critical piece of emergency info. Do list hormones, though.

When you list allergies, list only those that are true allergies, not simply side effects. For example, if you have been given morphine in the past and became nauseated that is *not* an allergy. If you had itching or facial swelling or shortness of breath, that *is* an allergy.

We don't really care about every little toenail surgery unless that is why you are in the emergency room. As physicians, we want to know about body-altering surgeries. Have you had your appendix out? Heart stints? Renal transplant? We don't need to know about your childhood broken bone.

If your emergency contact person is not a blood relative, be sure they have some legal note that they can be given your medical information. It is a good idea to have a medical power of attorney, if you can trust that person to act in your best interest. Do not give power over your life and death to someone who might want your estate more than you!

Also, write on the top of the form the date of latest update. That way if there are conflicts of information on different summary sheets, your doctor knows the latest version.

NAME_____ DOB_____ AGE_____

ADDRESS_____

EMERGENCY CONTACT OR NEXT OF KIN / CONTACT NO.

_____ PH_____

ALLERGY_____ CAUSES_____
_____ CAUSES_____
_____ CAUSES_____
_____ CAUSES_____
_____ CAUSES_____

ACTIVE MEDICAL PROBLEMS: SMOKING HISTORY:_____

1.

2.

3.

4.

5.

PAST SURGERY: _____

PRESCRIPTION MEDICATIONS:

1.   6.

2.   7.

3.   8.

4.   9.

5,   10.

OTHER ISSUES OF IMPORTANCE:

NOTES

CHAPTER 1: HOW WE GOT HERE

1. William Bruce Cameron, *Informal Sociology: A Casual Introduction to Sociological Thinking* (New York: Random House, 1963), 13.

2. *Lancet Oncology* 8 (2007): 784–96.

3. Public Health Agency of Canada, "Organized Breast Cancer Screening Programs in Canada: Report on Program Performance in 2001–2002."

4. Jeremy Laurance, "Dialysis Shortage Exposes Failings of NHS," *Independent* (UK), January 14, 2003.

5. A. A. Ray et al., "Waiting for Cardiac Surgery: Results of a Risk-Stratified Queuing Process," *Circulation* 104 (2001): 92–98.

6. Michael Pearson, "The VA's troubled history," *CNN Politics*, May 30, 2014, http://www.cnn.com/2014/05/23/politics/va-scandals-timeline/.

7. Craig Harris and Rob O'Dell, "Phoenix VA gave out $10 mil in bonuses in past 3 years," *AZ Central*, June 17, 2014, http://www.azcentral.com/story/news/arizona/investigations/2014/06/17/phoenix-va-gave-mil-bonuses-last-years/10653263/.

8. Sarah Kliff, "Screwed-up bonus payments are at the heart of the VA scandal," Vox, May 30, 2014, http://www.vox.com/2014/5/30/5762482/health-incentives-gone-wrong.

9. "A Survey of America's Physicians: Practice Patterns and Perspectives," Physicians Foundation, September 2012, http://www.physiciansfoundation.org/uploads/default/Physicians_Foundation_2012_Biennial_Survey.pdf.

10. Pamela Wible, MD, "What I've learned from saving physicians from suicide," *KevinMD*, a MedPage Today blog, May 27, 2013, http://www.kevinmd.com/blog/2013/05/learned-saving-physicians-suicide.html.

CHAPTER 2: THE COMING DOCTOR SHORTAGE

1. As an orthopaedic surgeon, I cannot resist recounting a little history. You will see we modern-day bone doctors referred to as orthopaedic or orthopedic surgeons—with or without the *a*. With the *a*, orthopaedic in Latin means "straight child," and that was the original meaning of the term when coined by Nicholas Andry in 1741. To spell it without the *a* means, in Latin, "straight foot"—and we are not just concerned with feet, so I pedantically insist on the *a*.

2. Ronald T. Libby, *The Criminalization of Medicine; America's War on Doctors* (Westport, CT: Praeger, 2007), 5, 9.

3. Personal communication with Jane Orient, MD, at the AAPS meeting in Denver Colorado 2013.

4. "Surgeon Reports to Prison; Government Sends Message," Association of American Physicians and Surgeons, December 11, 2012, http://www.aapsonline.org/index.php/site/article/surgeon_reports_to_prison_government_sends_message_states_aaps/.

5. "American College of Surgeons, "The Surgical Workforce in the United States: Profile and Recent Trends," 2010, http://www.acshpri.org/documents/ACSHPRI_Surgical_Workforce_in_US_apr2010.pdf.

CHAPTER 3: WHY YOUR DOCTOR IS OUT OF DATE

1. Casey Luskin, "Is There a 'Consensus' in Science? Remembering the Late Michael Crichton," Evolution News and Views, November 14, 2008, http://www.evolutionnews.org/2008/11/is_there_a_consensus_in_scienc013351.html.

2. Gordon C. S. Smith and Jill P. Pell, "Parachute use to prevent death and major trauma related to gravitational challenge: systematic review of randomised controlled trials," *BMJ* 327 (2003): 1459–61; http://www.neonatology.org/pdf/ParachuteUseRPCT.pdf.

CHAPTER 4: THE FINAL GOVERNMENT TAKEOVER

1. Perry Chiaramonte, "High cost of Common Core has states rethinking the national education standards," Fox News, February 05, 2014, http://www.foxnews.com/us/2014/02/05/number-states-backing-out-common-core-testing-maryland-schools-low-on-funding/.

2. Thomas J. DiLorenzo, "Our Totalitarian Regulatory Bureaucracy," *Mises Daily*, July 26, 2010, http://mises.org/daily/4585.

3. Bob Beauprez, "The Telescope: The Nationalization of the Banks," *A Line of Sight*, July 19, 2011, http://alos.thinkrootshq.com/policy/the-telescope-the-nationalization-of-the-banks.

4. See "Public Law 111 – 148 – Patient Protection and Affordable Care Act," on the website of the U.S. Government Printing Office, http://www.gpo.gov/fdsys/pkg/PLAW-111publ148/content-detail.html.

5. Clyde Wayne Crews Jr., *Ten Thousand Commandments 2012: An Annual Snapshot of the Federal Regulatory State*, Competitive Enterprise Institute, http://cei.org/10kc.

6. The Physicians Foundation, *A Survey of America's Physicians: Practice Patterns and Perspectives* (2012), http://www.physiciansfoundation.org/uploads/default/Physicians_Foundation_2012_Biennial_Survey.pdf, 11.

7. Kathryn Serkes, "Disheartened Doctors, Patient Problems: AAPS Biannual Survey of Physicians on Medicare and Patients' Access to Care," *Journal of American Physicians and Surgeons* 8, no. 4 (Winter 2003), http://www.jpands.org/vol8no4/serkes.pdf.

8. Govind Persad, Alan Wertheimer, and Ezekiel A. Immanuel, "Principles for Allocation of Scarce Medical Interventions," *Lancet* 373, no. 9661 (2009): 423–31.

9. Yuri N. Maltsev, "What Soviet Medicine Teaches Us," *Mises Daily*, June 22, 2012, http://mises.org/daily/3650.

10. Michael P. Coleman et al., "Cancer survival in five continents: a worldwide population-based study," *Lancet Oncology* 9, no. 8 (August 2008): 730–56, http://www.thelancet.com/journals/lanonc/issue/vol9no8/PIIS1470-2045(08)X7090-1.

CHAPTER 5: WHAT THE MELTDOWN WILL LOOK LIKE

1. Chad Terbune, "Closure of three Southland hospitals may be part of a trend," *Los Angeles Times*, April 3, 2013, http://articles.latimes.com/2013/apr/03/business/la-fi-pacific-hospitals-closing-20130404.

2. Suzanne Dion, RN, former Montreal nurse in personal communication to the author in 2005.

3. *Pogue* is a pejorative military term for a bureaucrat—someone who pushes paper but who does not share in the stress and risk of combat as a front-line soldier. This term desperately needs adoption into civilian life.

4. P. Sullivan, MD, oncologist, in personal communication to the author in 2007.

CHAPTER 8: DIET: WHAT SCIENCE REALLY TELLS US

1. From the motion picture *Vanilla Sky*, directed by Cameron Crowe (Paramount, 2001).

2. Doug A. Scott, "Serum Vitamin B$_{12}$ and Blood Cell Values in Vegetarians," *Annals of Nutrition and Metabolism* 26, no. 4 (1982): 209–16.

3. H-X Wang et al., "Vitamin B(12) and folate in relation to the development of Alzheimer's disease," *Neurology* 56, no. 9 (2001): 1188–94.

4. C. Lord et al., "Dietary animal protein intake: association with muscle mass index in older women," *Journal of Nutrition, Health & Aging* 11, no. 5 (2007): 383–87.

5. T. A. Outila et al., "Dietary intake of vitamin D in premenopausal, healthy vegans was insufficient to maintain concentrations of serum 25-hydroxyvitamin D and intact parathyroid hormone within normal ranges during the winter in Finland," *Journal of the American Dietetic Association* 100, no. 4 (2000): 434–41.

6. M. Ureshima et al., "Randomized trial of vitamin D supplementation to prevent seasonal influenza A in schoolchildren," *American Journal of Clinical Nutrition* 91, no. 5 (2010):1255–60.

7. Federico Carbone and Fabrizio Montecucco, "The Role of the Intraplaque Vitamin D System in Atherogenesis," *Scientifica*, November 18, 2013, http://www.hindawi.com/journals/scientifica/2013/620504/.

8. T. Shoji et al, "Lower risk for cardiovascular mortality in oral alpha-hydroxy vitamin D$_3$ users in a haemodialysis population," *Nephrology, Dialysis, Transplant* 19, no. 1 (January 2004): 179–84, http://www.ncbi.nlm.nih.gov/pubmed/14671054.

9. C. F. Garland et al., "Breast Cancer Risk according to Serum 25 Hydroxy Vitamin D; Meta-analysis of Dose Response" (abstract), American Association of Cancer Research Annual Meeting (2008).

10. Inge Everaert et al., "Vegetarianism, female gender and increasing age, but not *CNDP1* genotype, are associated with reduced muscle carnosine levels in humans," *Springer Link* 40, no. 4 (April 2011): 1221–29.

11. "Serum sex hormones and endurance performance after a lacto-ovo vegetarian and a mixed diet," *Medicine & Science in Sports and Exercise* 24, no. 11 (1992):1290–97.

12. Lierre Keith, *The Vegetarian Myth: Food, Justice, and Sustainability* (Oakland, CA: PM Press, 2009), 92. Similarly, a short article by Dr. Stephen Byrnes, titled "Myths & Truths About Vegetarianism" and posted on the website of the Weston A. Price Foundation, outlines the perils and mistaken thinking about vegetarianism. See http://www.westonaprice.org/health-topics/abcs-of-nutrition/myths-of-vegetarianism/.

13. Gary Taubes, *Good Calories, Bad Calories: Fats, Carbs, and the Controversial Science of Diet and Health*, (New York: Anchor, 2008).

14. See Brian S. Peskin and Robert Jay Rowen, *PEO Solution: Conquering Cancer, Diabetes and Heart Disease with Parent Essential Oils* (Pinnacle, 2015), available at http://www.peo-solution.com/. See also http://www.peskinprotocol.com/supplements/peos.htm.

15. Patrick L. McGeer, Michael Schulzer, and Edith G. McGeer, "Arthritis and anti-inflammatory agents as possible protective factors for Alzheimer's disease," *Neurology* 47, no. 2 (August 1996): 425–32.

16. R. M. Murray, J. G. Greene, and J. H. Adams, "Analgesic Abuse and Dementia," *Lancet* 298, no. 7718 (July 21, 1971).

17. G. R. N. Jones, "Causes of Alzheimer's disease: paracetamol (acetaminophen) today? Amphetamines tomorrow?" *Medical Hypotheses* 56, no. 1 (January 2001): 121–23, http://www.ncbi.nlm.nih.gov/pubmed/11133268.

18. National Survey on Drug Use and Health, 2010, http://www.samhsa.gov/data/NSDUH/2012SummNatFindDetTables/NationalFindings/NSDUHresults2012.htm#ch3.1.

19. R. O. Roberts et al., "Relative Intake of Macronutrients Impacts Risk of Mild Cognitive Impairment or Dementia," *Journal of Alzheimer's Disease* 32, no. 2 (2012): 329–39.

20. Rebecca West et al., "Better Memory Functioning Associated with Higher Total and Low density Lipoprotein Cholesterol Levels in Very Elderly Subjects without the Apolipoprotein e4 Alletel," *American Journal of Geriatric Psychiatry* 16, no. 9 (2008): 781–85; cited in David Perlmutter, *Grain Brain: The Surprising Truth about Wheat, Carbs, and Sugar—Your Brain's Silent Killers*, with Kristin Loberg (New York: Little, Brown, 2013), 74.

21. L. M. de Lau et al., "Serum Cholesterol Levels and the Risk of Parkinson's Disease," *American Journal of Epidemiology* 164, no. 10 (2006): 998–1002.

22. Probably the best summary of a good diet is found on the website of the Weston A. Price Foundation. See Jill Nienhiser, "Dietary Guidelines," January 1, 2000, http://www.westonaprice.org/health-topics/abcs-of-nutrition/dietary-guidelines/.

CHAPTER 11: PREPARING YOURSELF: SUPPLEMENTS

1. Chris Kresser, "How too much Omega-6 and not enough Omega-3 is making us sick," Chris Kresser blog, http://chriskresser.com/how-too-much-omega-6-and-not-enough-omega-3-is-making-us-sick.

2. Barry Sears, *The Anti-Inflammation Zone: Reversing the Silent Epidemic That's Destroying Our Health* (New York: Regan, 2005).

CHAPTER 15: BE YOUR OWN CORPSMAN: STORING AND STOCKPILING MEDICINES

1. Robbe C. Lyon et al., "Stability Profiles of Drug Products Extended beyond Labeled Expiration Dates," *Journal of Pharmaceutical Sciences* 95, no. 7 (July 2006): 1549–60, available at http://onlinelibrary.wiley.com/doi/10.1002/jps.20636/abstract.

2. Medication Safety, Safe Kids Worldwide website, accessed July 24, 2014, http://www.safekids.org/medicinesafety.

CHAPTER 16: STOCKPILING AND DISTRIBUTING SUPPLIES

1. Ethan A. Huff, "Border Patrol agents being widely infected with diseases; union VP warns all of America at risk," *Natural News*, July 17, 2014, http://www.naturalnews.com/046030_illegal_immigration_infectious_diseases_Border_Patrol_agents.html.

CHAPTER 17: REAL EMERGENCIES CAN'T WAIT

1. Centers for Disease Control and Prevention, Rabies, "Other Animals," accessed July 25, 2014, www.cdc.gov/rabies/exposure/animals/other.html.

2. "Prevention of Rabies in Humans: Bats in Buildings—Investigative Steps," accessed July 25, 2014, http://epi.publichealth.nc.gov/cd/lhds/manuals/rabies/docs/bats_in_bldgs.pdf.

CHAPTER 20: COLDS AND FLU-LIKE SYMPTOMS

1. New Recommended Daily Amounts of Calcium and Vitamin D, NIH Medicine Plus, 2011, http://www.nlm.nih.gov/medlineplus/magazine/issues/winter11/articles/winter11pg12.html.

2. *Anti-aging medicine* refers to that subspecialty of medicine focusing on prolonging quality and length of life through the use of avant-garde techniques based on the latest science.

CHAPTER 21: BITES

1. A good photo resource is http://www.medicinenet.com/black_widow_brown_recluse_pictures_slideshow/article.htm.

CHAPTER 28: DENTAL CARE

1. See Lee Hieb, "Fluoride: 1 More Deadly Government Experiment," WND, March 4, 2013, http://www.wnd.com/2013/03/fluoride-1-more-deadly-government-experiment/.

CHAPTER 29: THE FUTURE OF MEDICINE

1. T. S. Eliot, "The Hollow Men" (1925).

INDEX